....

Praise for *Cook Food*

....

Overwhelmed by all the politics on your plate? Paralyzed by guilt every time you shop for food? In this delectable guide, Lisa Jervis shows not just how easy it can be to eat with your conscience and with the planet, but also how cheap, how swift, and how delightful it is to feel at home in the kitchen. −Raj Patel, author of *Stuffed and Starved: The Hidden Battle for the World Food System*

With a heavy emphasis on local and unprocessed eating, *Cook Food* will help you overcome your hesitations about going veg or passing on the vegan bologna. A great resource for those stepping into the kitchen for the first time and vegetarians who want to go the distance to make this a healthier planet. −Siue Moffat, author of *Lickin' the Beaters: Low Fat Vegan Desserts*

Want an opportunity to make the world better several times a day? Learn to feed yourself using the rational, witty, simple, and ethical guidelines in Lisa Jervis's manual, *Cook Food*. It's the Dennis Kucinich of cookbooks: petite, political, powerful, with a profound lack of B.S. Read it and eat. −Jennifer Baumgardner, coauthor of *Manifesta: Young Women, Feminism, and the Future* and author of *Look Both Ways: Bisexual Politics*.

Cook Food is equal parts inspiration, call to arms, cooking school, and guide to making everything more yummy. It also demonstrates, powerfully, how to marry important ideals about food with the realities of day-to-day living. —Rabbi Danya Ruttenberg, author of *Surprised By God: How I Learned to Stop Worrying and Love Religion*

Finally! A thoroughly smart and useful book on the topic of food and social justice that fat people (and people of all sizes) can enjoy. Lisa offers so very many good, convincing reasons to make a smaller footprint that it's clear we can discard as unnecessary all of those arguments made on the backs of fat people. Thank you, Lisa, for a delicious, truly cruelty-free book! —Marilyn Wann, author of *FAT!SO?—Because You Don't Have to Apologize for Your Size!*

Lisa Jervis's head, heart, and taste buds are all so exactly in the right place, and reading *Cook Food* is like having her in your kitchen with you. This book feels like a strong, sane, healthy, funny friend, chatting with you while you cook and saying "try a pinch of that." It may well prove to be just the kind of companionship people need in order to make that step toward really changing the way they shop, cook, eat, and think about food. —Thisbe Nissen, author of *The Ex-Boyfriend Cookbook* and *Osprey Island*

With good humor and a level head, this little treatise strips the elitism and the nutrition-fascism out of fresh, honest, vegetable-centric food, and offers robust, immensely usable recipes to teach and inspire both the whole-foods newbie and the experienced cook. —Hanne Blank, author of *Virgin: The Untouched History* and *Unruly Appetites*

Lisa Jervis has convinced me that I can be a great cook. We can't come close to being perfect when it comes to preserving the planet or our health, but this persuasive, friendly, and usable book gives us the impetus to be the best we can. We can't change the world overnight, but we can change our eating habits. −Amy Richards, author of *Opting In: Having A Child Without Losing Yourself* and cofounder of Third Wave Foundation.

Cook Food is an informative, accessible, and downright fun guide to cooking healthily, locally, and responsibly. In addition to the many tasty recipes, Lisa Jervis demystifies the kitchen experience by explaining basic cooking tools and techniques, and encouraging improvisation. A must-have for progressive-minded foodies everywhere! −Julia Serano, author of *Whipping Girl: A Transsexual Woman on Sexism and the Scapegoating of Femininity*

Sure, I appreciate a cookbook with a social conscience. Plus, on a very practical level, *Cook Food* is just useful to have around. But, hands down, I most value this book for its sense of flavor. Lisa Jervis serves up simple yet sophisticated taste combinations with a global flare that make it easy−and even fun−to do the right thing with one's diet. −Paula Kamen, author of *Feminist Fatale* and *Finding Iris Chang*

Cook Food

a manualfesto for
easy, healthy, local eating

Lisa Jervis

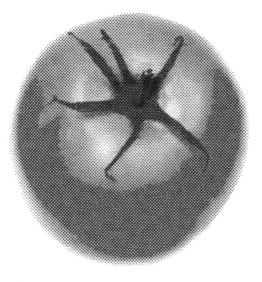

Cook Food: A Manualfesto for Easy, Healthy, Local Eating
By Lisa Jervis

ISBN: 978-1-60486-073-3
Library of Congress Control Number: 2009901376
Copyright © 2009 Lisa Jervis
This edition copyright © 2009 PM Press
All Rights Reserved

PM Press
PO Box 23912
Oakland, CA 94623
www.pmpress.org

Book & cover design by Benjamin Shaykin
Author photo by Drew Beck
Printed in the USA on recycled paper.

to my mother

....

who taught me how to be at home in the kitchen

contents

what's this book all about?
(a.k.a., introduction)

IN A NUTSHELL, THIS BOOK IS AN ATTEMPT TO MAKE LIFE easier for people who want to cook and eat healthy homemade food without spending a ton of time and money. But that's not all it is.

It could also be described as an attempt to provide some basic tools for people who want to be healthier and lighten the footprint of the way they eat by emphasizing whole foods (meaning unprocessed things, not the union-busting grocery chain), local ingredients, and cooking without animal products.

It could be seen as a call to action against our wasteful, unjust, destructive, unhealthy, industrialized, corporate-dominated food system (with recipes).

It could just be a vegan-friendly* cookbook. Or a quick-cooking cookbook. Or an improvisational cookbook. Or a farmers market cookbook.

Or an overly complicated way to get my friends to stop asking me to tell them how I made the dinner we're eating.

....

* I emphasize cooking without animal products—there's nothing in this book that isn't vegan as the recipe is written, with no substituting necessary—but sometimes I do suggest possible cheese or egg additions to a dish. And I believe in using only vegan ingredients when they are totally equivalent to their non-vegan

To synthesize all those things, this book is a short, quirky education in simple cooking; healthy, light-footprint eating; and the politics of food.

It is also, and I can't stress this enough, totally flexible. All the recipes are approximate (except the two for baked goods, 'cause though the flavors in there are substitutable, the proportions of flour, oil, etc. are not). If you're not crazy about any ingredient or flavor, use less of it than I call for (or eliminate it altogether). If you love it, use more. If you like an ingredient or flavor that I don't call for, and you think it would be good in whatever is it you're making, throw it on in there. If there's a vegetable listed that you don't have in the house, but you do have something else, make a swap. Experiment, try new things, make the recipes your own. Cooking is about principles and techniques, not rigid ingredients and directions. Trust your instincts. If you've done any amount of cooking before—or even if you haven't, because, no matter what, you've doubtless done plenty of eating—you already have a sense of what'll be good. Something as simple as your knowledge of what you like to eat, combined with the simple tools in this book (see "Tips and Techniques," page 39) will guide you to a good meal with any ingredients and flavors you like.

So what does that mean, "healthy, light-footprint eating"?

The concept of a light footprint is one I stole from other sustainability conversations because I think it most accurately describes what I'm aiming for with my food choices, which can't be ade-

....

counterparts (e.g., olive oil is just as good if not better for sautéing the base of your bean stew as butter is), or easily substitutable (so many baked goods don't actually need eggs or butter to work). But a carefully sourced and thoughtfully chosen cheese to adorn your meal is irreplaceable and can be a beautiful thing.

quately or accurately described with words like "vegan" or "vegetarian." Basically, I'm trying to be as healthy as I can and minimize my negative impact on the environment and on other beings. So I try to choose foods that are locally produced, minimally packaged, minimally processed, and organic whenever possible. I avoid sweets and junk food (most of the time—I'm only human, after all). I source my animal products very carefully. It's a lot easier to say "I'm a healthy, light-footprint eater" than it is to say "Well, I try to avoid white flour, refined sugar, and hydrogenated things; I buy a huge percentage of my food at the farmers market; and although I'm not vegetarian or vegan I stay away from animal products unless I know where they came from and under what conditions the animals lived." Because I buy almost all my fruits and vegetables at the farmers market, I'm always eating in season, and everything else (grains, tofu, nuts, spices, beans, etc.) comes from a local independent grocery store with a great bulk section.

As to why I wanted to write a whole (short) book about it—well, obviously it's about a lot more than just what I choose to eat for dinner. Food politics have become a pretty hot topic over the last few years, what with writers like Eric Schlosser, Michael Pollan, Marion Nestle, Raj Patel, and many others exploring and explaining the effects of industrialized food on individuals, communities, and the natural world—not to mention news events like salmonella-tainted spinach and tomatoes, melamine-tainted milk and eggs, meat recalls, and popcorn-factory workers getting lung disease from artificial-butter fumes. So it's likely you know this already, but just in case you don't: The average bite of food travels 1,500 miles from where it's grown to where it is eaten. Monoculture crops and centralized food distribution vastly increase the likelihood of outbreaks of foodborne illnesses (as Michael Pollan put it in the October 15, 2006, issue of the *New York Times Magazine*, the fact that a single facility can produce so much bagged spinach means that "we're washing the whole nation's salad in one big sink"). U.S. farm subsidies benefit massive corporate farmers using huge amounts of chemical inputs on their monoculture crops—much of which will be processed into animal feed, high-fructose corn syrup, and other products of dubious value—at the expense of small farmers growing food that can be eaten, by people, without further ado. These subsidies enable the packaged food that fills the middle of the supermarket and derives its nutrition, if it has any at all, from vitamins added back in after they've been stripped out in processing. Too many low-income neighborhoods have no supermarkets at all, leaving residents without access to fresh produce, period, let alone any that's local or organic. Farmworkers often labor under dangerous conditions for very little pay. With only a few hard-to-find exceptions, animals are raised for food on factory farms under hideous conditions. In short, the current U.S. food system—which, through globalization and other related forces, reverberates worldwide—has been designed and built by agribusiness to maximize profits. People who eat food and live with the consequences of this system, not to mention the animals that are used for food by those of us who choose to eat meat, eggs, and dairy products, lose big. Not to be too hippy-dippy about it, but when you widen the lens even further to include ecosystem health, it really means that every single living being on the planet is affected.

Translating all this information into decisions about what to eat is extra-complicated, because environmental concerns, labor issues, animal welfare, what's best for your own health, what you can afford, and what you can get at your neighborhood market don't always line up neatly. When I'm faced with a food choice, whether I'm at the store, at the farmers market, or at a restaurant, the issues I care about often conflict with each other. Some choices are relatively obvious. Superficial affordability is the only positive thing about a fast-food burger with a slice of cardboard tomato on a white flour bun that's loaded with dough conditioners and probably high-fructose corn syrup to boot: It's a low-quality food produced with lots of pesticides, hormones, and antibiotics under terrible working conditions for both humans and animals, plus food additives aplenty. And it tastes kinda gross. But affordability can be damn powerful—even if it's dependent on masking the true cost of food production by exploiting workers and damaging the environment.

What about fake meats made from soy and wheat? There's no question they're better from the simplest animal-welfare perspective, but they're highly processed and usually heavily packaged, so they aren't that healthy for me and aren't as much better for the environment as I might hope. (The waste in packaging and the industrial processing—plus the probable sourcing of ingredients produced by huge monoculture agribusiness farms—mean that being lower on the food chain doesn't mean as much as it should.) They're unknown but probably better on the labor front, if only because slaughterhouses are one of the most dangerous places in the world to work, period.

And what about tofu and tempeh? Some folks believe that the estrogens in soy contribute to elevated cancer risk; the health benefits of soy touted by food and nutraceutical companies are certainly overblown. Then there's the deforestation, displacement of rural populations, pesticide use, genetic modification, and other ugliness involved in soy farming. But I eat both tofu and tempeh regularly and without worry, and I continue to recommend them. Here's why: They're very whole and unprocessed compared to the soy in packaged foods, so if you're avoiding those, you can eat other soy without overloading your body with it. More important, the yield of the multinational, monoculture-based soy production industry that's wreaking such global havoc goes almost entirely to animal feed, food additives, and biofuels. The consumption of tofu and tempeh is miniscule compared to that, so I strongly believe that if I'm swapping animal protein out of my diet for relatively unprocessed soy, I'm doing all right.

Humanely produced organic cheese and eggs from the farmers market seem pretty great all around, but am I letting myself be lulled into overconsumption of animal products by the bucolic pictures of grazing goats and pecking chickens posted at the booths? Meat carries the same questions, but more seriously, because, duh, it involves an actual death. Is indulging my cravings okay just because I can make chili from ground meat that came from one cow, and the guy selling it to me can tell me exactly where and how the cow lived and what it ate? What if I believe those cravings involve not taste or whim but a serious nutritional need? And if that's true, what should I do when a nutritional need hits at a time when I can't budget for organic, pasture-raised meat?

To top it all off, I know that my easy access to good grocery stores and affordable farmers markets is a luxury that most people just don't have, and that what I define as affordable is far from universal. By focusing so much on my individual choices, am I neglecting—or even obscuring—the key issues of food access?

All these questions mean I could—and sometimes do, unfortunately—spend a lot of time with my mental wheels spinning. Oy.

In the end, we can all only do the best we can. Which actually means a lot.

Wait, back up a minute. How do you define "healthy"?

To me, the less processed something is, the more healthy it is. But other than that—which basically entails cooking a lot, avoiding most snack foods that come in boxes or bags, and carefully reading the label of anything I'm thinking about buying—I don't worry too much about my nutritional needs. I think it's not only a waste of time but seriously bad for your mental health to worry about incorporating a checklist of micronutrients into your diet based on the latest medical studies or food-industry health claims. (See Michael Pollan's article about this phenomenon, dubbed "nutritionism," in the January 28, 2007, issue of the *New York Times Magazine*; it's available online and it's also an excerpt from his stellar book *In Defense of Food*.) If you cook for yourself with fresh ingredients and you don't eat the same thing every day, you're damn likely to keep your nutritional bases covered. That's healthy.

I also don't worry about fat and salt, two delicious and useful substances that have been unfairly demonized by certain sectors of the food and nutrition establishment. They make your food taste good, and you shouldn't be afraid of them.** Be skeptical of all those medical warnings against salt and fat. In my opinion, a lot of health issues that have been blamed on salt and fat in general are

....

** If you have a specific health condition that is related to fat or salt, then of course pay attention to that. For instance, if you have salt-sensitive high blood pressure, then yeah, you have to eat a low-salt diet.

actually caused by processed foods that contain very specific kinds of fat (cough, hydrogenated oils, cough) and happen to be salty.

Okay, but what do you mean by "processed"?

Good question. There are actually two very different ways the term "processing" can be understood when it comes to food. The first meaning is totally benign; it just refers to anything that must be done to food in order to make it ready to eat. In its simplest form, this means things like removing inedible plant parts like husks, shells, hulls, and peels; chopping; and cooking. In that sense, you process food yourself every time you make a meal. Some forms of necessary and nondestructive processing are a little more complicated: canning and preserving, making cheese and yogurt, grinding grains into flour, etc. You probably don't choose to do these things at home, but you could if you wanted to (and see "Further Resources," page 117, for more information on that).

The second meaning, the one I'm talking about when I'm talking about avoiding processed food, is the kind of processing that transforms a raw ingredient into something else entirely, either by removing some edible part of it, chemically treating it, or isolating one element of it and tossing everything else (or turning the other elements into some other food additive). This ranges from the relatively uncomplicated but still nutritionally bankrupt removal of bran and germ that yields white flour to the intense industrial processes that make high-fructose corn syrup, hydrogenated oils, lecithin, and things listed on ingredient labels as "natural flavors," which are anything but.

It's pretty easy to tell the difference between good processed food and bad processed food. Benignly processed food generally has few ingredients (a can of tomatoes has tomatoes, salt, and sometimes one other preservative item), which are all pronounceable and generally recognizable as food (unlike, say, disodium guanylate or yellow 6 lake). You can make it at home in your own kitchen if you have enough time, energy, and knowledge (and yes, if you wanted to crush soybeans at home, you could make both tofu and tempeh).

Then there are some things that are somewhere in the middle: cornstarch, soy sauce, many oils, etc.–these are really useful in the kitchen and I feel good about them, even though they aren't actually whole foods. They're not *that* processed, and, as you might have guessed, I come down on the side of ease a lot of the time. Once cooking and eating guidelines meant to make your life better become overly restrictive, they start to do the opposite of what they should. Which leads naturally to what I expect might be your next question.

Realistically, is it really possible to eat local, unprocessed, animal-free food all the time?

All the time? Like, every part of every meal? No. Like I said before, we can all only do the best we can. One-hundred-percent local diets aren't realistic for anyone (no one should try to cook without spices!), and even mostly local diets are inaccessible for many; no one should run the risk of scurvy in the wintertime if they don't have a huge freezer and/or countless free hours in the late summer to spend canning. Time, energy, money, climate, individual nutritional needs, and how much you like to cook and think about food all affect what you can do. The point is to fit a healthy, humane, and–don't forget–pleasurable eating style comfortably into your life.

Sounds like a lot of trouble.

Well, yeah, sometimes it is. But I think it's worth it. My personal story of why goes a little something like this:

Several years ago, in line with the larger culture's emerging critique of processed food and industrial agriculture, I was cutting down my sugar consumption and learning more about the evils of things like hydrogenation, shipping vegetables around the globe, food additives, and factory farming. At the same time, I had a new coworker who was superhardcore in her commitment to veganism and whole foods. We started talking endlessly about the politics and ethics of food choices (and the connections between those politics and seemingly unrelated social justice movements), the health benefits of unrefined food, what looked best at the farmers market, and tasty cooking ideas.

Then another friend issued a challenge: We would do the veganish whole-foods-only thing for a month, cooking and eating together and keeping each other on track, and he would never eat fast food again, ever. So for one month I ate no white flour, no refined sugar, almost nothing packaged at all. My life filled up with lots of brown rice, beans, roasted vegetables, and tofu stir-fries. I couldn't go entirely, strictly vegan, even for only a month, but the only non-vegan thing I ate was yogurt. (I knew I couldn't live like that forever, but I knew I could hack it for four weeks.) Every Sunday my friend would come over, along with a few others, and we would each cook something healthy and share the results to eat throughout the week.

The potluck afternoons were great fun, but even better was how I felt mentally and physically. I had more energy in general and more stamina throughout the workday. No sugar meant no sugar crashes and fewer headaches. I was usually fully satisfied by my meals rather than casting about afterwards for something to make me feel truly done eating. My mood also improved, though I don't know whether it was related to the diet change itself or my newly higher energy levels. As hard as it was to give up the sourdough from my favorite local bakery and the Cheez-Its and Twizzlers I would eat in front of the TV or at the movies, I knew I could never go back to my old ways. Just not getting that midafternoon need-to-put-my-head-down-on-my-desk-and-nap feeling was enough to keep me focused on putting good things into by body. Sure, the sweet tooth was—and still is—a real issue, but I discovered that the less sugar I ate, the less I wanted it. My palate really changed; things that I used to love started to taste way too sweet and/or chemical-filled. Plus, I was living more in line with my political values, which always feels good.

I don't want to make it sound like I'm this paragon of brown-rice-eating self-righteous ethical-food perfectionism. I'm not. I indulge my junk food cravings when I really want to, and I end up eating cheese of unknown provenance much more often than I'd like to admit, especially when I'm eating out. I go through periods of meat cravings, and I heed them because I think they have nutritional significance. But, like I said, I do the best I can.

I'm on a tight budget. Can I really do this?

Yes. While fresh fruits and vegetables can seem expensive, when you think about how many servings of high-quality nutrition you can get out of an onion, a bunch of kale, a sweet potato, two cans of beans, a can of tomatoes, some spices, and some rice, you're doing pretty well on the budget front. A breakfast of steel-cut oats with a small handful of dried fruit, some nuts, and some olive oil costs about the same as a bowl of processed cereal with milk. Processed foods may be cheap per calorie, but they're expensive per unit of nutrition. And when you buy fresh food, you're paying only for food, not for packaging and marketing. It's still hard to beat fast-food "value" prices, I know, but making food yourself, especially when it means you can have leftovers to eat for lunch the next day, really is cost-effective.

Sure, some kinds of produce—cherries, blueberries, artichokes, and asparagus spring to mind—are always spendy. But greens (kale, collards, spinach, chard), potatoes (sweet and regular), broccoli and cauliflower, carrots, beets, green beans, and squash (both summer and winter) are widely available and generally affordable. Plus, fruits and veggies are always cheaper when they're in season than when they're not, so buying what's growing near you right now can save you money.

Organic food does cost more, and though I think it's well worth it—it's safer for workers, better for soil and water, healthier for eaters, and usually just plain tastes better—sometimes it's just not possible to spend extra. You can pick and choose what you spring for and what you don't: The so-called dirty dozen, the stuff that's most important to buy organic because the conventional versions are most contaminated, includes nectarines, peaches, pears, celery, apples, cherries, strawberries, grapes, spinach, potatoes, bell peppers, and raspberries. (Google "dirty dozen vegetables" if you want to know more.)

Meat, dairy, and eggs, if you choose to eat them, are definitely going to be much more expensive in their organic/sustainable/humane versions. This is *not* the place to skimp. Animal products are seriously contaminated by any antibiotics and pesticides used in their production, their environmental effects are horrendous, and the animal-treatment issues are pretty obvious. I don't like to get directive, and everyone's nutritional needs are different, but, if at all possible, it's so much better to lighten your budgetary load by eating more beans, soy, and nuts than it is to buy cheap meat.

Sounds like you're kinda spoiled by living in the foodcentric and year-round-growing-season-tastic Bay Area, and in a neighborhood that's well-served by grocery stores and farmers markets to boot. What about those of us without that kind of access?

Guilty as charged. First of all, see "Further Resources," page 117, for more information about finding food sources, getting involved in organizing to improve community access to fresh food, and growing your own food.

Second, again, you can do the best you can. Even if you live in a climate where the ground is frozen half the year, you can still eat seasonally, skipping tomatoes and strawberries in January and going with apples and root veggies instead, which keep for a long time and, even if they have to be trucked in from somewhere else, are probably coming from closer than, say, Chile. (Of course, there's the whole canning thing. Preserving food at home is not for everyone, but it's a great strategy for extending the availability of local produce, and it can also be pretty fun. I've got information about that in "Further Resources," too.)

So what now?

Read over the parts of the book that interest you. For those totally new to the kitchen, I've included some tips on stocking the pantry and what equipment you need; I've are also laid out some methods and principles that should be useful for both new and experienced cooks. Or you can skip any more reading, pick a recipe, and make yourself some dinner.

what you need in your cabinets and on your pot rack

I LOVE KITCHEN EQUIPMENT TO AN EMBARRASSING degree, whether we're talkin' pots and pans, gadgets, or countertop appliances. But I'm also all about thriftiness, and I realize that not everyone can or wants to spend hir hard-earned paycheck on 10-piece cookware sets or graters meant for one ingredient only. So I'm putting them into categories by necessity—and keep in mind that thrift shops can be kitchenware treasure troves. There are only two areas where quality is *really* important. The first is with pots and pans. Look for heavy bottoms, no warping (if you're buying used), no nonstick surface (it's been discovered that nonstick surfaces can off-gas toxic fumes into your food at high temperatures), and materials other than plain aluminum, which can too-easily leach harmful metal into your food (however, aluminum that has gone through a process called anodization is stable and great to cook with, so anodized aluminum cookware gets a thumbs-up from me). The second is knives. Skip the thrift store, ask for advice at the kitchenware store, and test the feel of different knives in your hand. For everything else, what you can find at Goodwill or on sale at whatever housewares store suits you is going to be just fine. If any of these items are unfamiliar or confusing to you, a Google image search should clarify things better than any description I could give. Also, you should know that this is a quirky list that suits how I cook. I use my microplane zester weekly but haven't touched my box grater in more than a year, so I consider the latter much less important. You'll doubtless need to make your own adjustments.

You can't really cook anything without these things:

- One good chef's knife (this can mean spending at least $60, but if you can swing it, you'll be glad you did)
- At least two good cutting boards (plastic, wood, or bamboo, your choice); you need two because no matter how good you are at scrubbing, the smell of garlic and onions will never quite come out—and you want to have one board that never touches them, so when you make fruit salad, you can make sure it has no garlic flavor
- A saucepan, a stockpot, or a sauté pan
- A baking sheet or low-sided roasting pan (see page 76 for more about this)
- A wooden spoon
- A heat-proof spatula
- A big mixing bowl
- A set of measuring cups and spoons
- A can opener
- A kitchen timer if your oven doesn't have one (though if you have a cell phone, you're probably carrying a timer in your pocket, so you can use that)
- A colander

Either you'll find it pretty frustrating, you'll be limited in what you can cook, or your food won't turn out as well if you don't also have:

- A saucepan, a stockpot, *and* a sauté pan
- A skillet or a griddle pan
- A paring knife or other knife smaller than a chef's knife
- A couple more wooden spoons
- At least one rubber spatula
- A ladle
- A microplane for zesting citrus
- A high-sided baking pan (such as a 9×9×4 pan used for the brownies on page 109)
- A few more mixing bowls of different sizes

These are also good to have around if you think you'll use them, and they're generally pretty reasonably priced (except the griddle pan, but if you're like me you'll use it all the time):

- A skillet *and* a griddle pan (mine is square and has a rim that's barely raised; I don't think I would use it as much if it were shaped differently or had higher sides)
- A steamer basket (you can always steam things in a shallow pool of water right in the pan, but these are under $10 new and practically given away in thrift stores)
- A box grater
- A citrus reamer
- A porcelain ginger grater (unless you hate ginger, duh)
- A stick blender (great for soups, smoothies, and whatnot, and so easy to clean)

- Spring-loaded tongs
- A pastry brush (for brushing the tops of things with oil)
- An oven thermometer (unless you don't plan to bake or roast; see the discussion of roasting, page 76)

If you plan to bake, you also need:
- Parchment paper (I also like silicone baking mats, but they're pricey and only worth it if you're going to use them all the time)
- A cooling rack or two
- Two or three more cookie sheets
- Muffin tins and/or a loaf pan or two
- A hand mixer
- A kitchen scale (worth the money if you're going to bake a lot, since most good baking recipes give quantities of flour and other dry ingredients in weight rather than volume, since it's more accurate; if you're only going to bake a little, skip it)

These are pricey, but seriously worth it:
- A rice cooker with a permanently attached hinged lid that clicks closed (you can get a cheaper one with a lift-off lid, but it won't cook your grains evenly without burning them or keep them warm without drying them out); I use mine at least once a day. You can make any kind of grain in them, not just rice, and if you also get one with a porridge setting, you can make oatmeal and experiment with oatmeal-like breakfasts using other grains (see "Nonrecipe Recipes," page 113). There are two major benefits of rice cookers over sticking a saucepan on a burner: The first is that you don't have to watch it, adjust the heat, or worry about when it's done; the appliance does all that for you, clicking over automatically

from "cooking" to "keep warm." The second is the "keep warm" setting itself–you can make breakfast the night before, or make part of your dinner in the morning before you go to work–or you can just have a steady supply of hot grains on hand. Rice cookers come in sizes ranging from four cups (ideal if you cook mostly for yourself only) to 12 (great if you feed six or more people at once on a regular basis). You'll probably need to spend between $100 and $125 for a new good one (the crappy lift-off lid ones can be as cheap as $30), but friends (and Craigslist) can be a great source of deals on stuff like this.

• A food processor; the only recipes in this book that use one are the sauces, so it may seem odd that I'm recommending one. But I am, 'cause I really believe in how useful they are. It's an investment of about a hundred bucks, and once you have it, you'll find yourself using it for all sorts of things you never thought about before.

I don't recommend:
• A garlic press (it's almost as easy and way better to chop, plus those suckers are hell to clean)
• A wok, unless your burners get really hot and you're serious about Chinese cooking
• A microwave oven (they cost a lot, take up space, and don't do anything that you can't do another way)
• A blender other than a stick blender (food processors are more versatile, plus they're generally more effective for any task your stick blender can't handle)

what you need in your pantry, refrigerator, and spice rack

ONE OF THE KEYS TO BEING ABLE TO COOK UP A TASTY MEAL quickly is having the necessary ingredients in the house already. Here are my suggestions for stocking your kitchen. Though my lists are also useful for making things that aren't addressed in this book, I'm assuming that you're going to be cooking the recipes in here. So, especially when it comes to herbs and spices, I've made no attempt to be exhaustive; you should of course be stocking anything that you like and/or think you'll use. And as with everything else, if you don't like the flavor of any item, just ignore my advice to buy it. Buy organic if and when you can, and always look for expeller-pressed and/or cold-pressed oils (other extraction processes involve chemical solvents, yuck). The key to an affordable pantry is finding a place to buy spices in bulk–it can be the difference between paying $4 or 50¢ for a couple ounces of cumin.

You need these in your pantry or fridge, and they last forever:
- Assorted dried or canned beans* (such as black, kidney, pinto,

* Dried beans are cheaper than canned beans and, since they're available in bulk and go through less processing (you're essentially processing them yourself when you soak and cook them), they also have a lighter footprint. And, depending

garbanzo, cannelini; if you're using canned, look for low-salt versions so you can control your own seasoning)

• Brown rice

• Canned diced tomatoes** (look for low-salt versions so you can control your own seasoning; also avoid ones with added basil or other flavors for the same reason)

• Canola or grapeseed oil*** (it's always good to have a neutral oil on hand for things where olive has too strong a flavor)

....

on where you're shopping, you can often find more variety—including interesting and unusual heirlooms—when you're in the market for dried beans. So dried beans are freakin' great. But I have to be honest, I hardly ever cook with them, which is why my recipes call for cans. The extra step of presoaking and the much longer cooking time means that you really need to plan ahead, and that's just not realistic for me most of the time—and I'm thinkin' it's not that realistic for you, either, since you're reading this book on healthy convenience cooking. So by all means go for dried beans if you can fit them into your schedule. But don't let avoidance of cans stop you from eating the tasty, healthy, affordable, animal-free staple that is beans.

** Tomatoes are the only vegetable I recommend buying in cans. There are a few reasons for this: They're necessary to get the best flavor from certain dishes; the canned version works well in those dishes, sometimes even better than fresh; and those dishes are often most appealing in winter, when fresh tomatoes are out of season anyway. (That doesn't mean they're not available—tomatoes are probably the most common and affordable out-of-season produce item. But winter supermarket tomatoes are vile and flavorless. You're better off putting cotton balls in your stew. Just say no.)

*** Canola oil does have some potential problems. First of all, all non-organic canola available in North America is pretty much guaranteed to be genetically modified, and even the organic stuff may be contaminated with GM material. In the face of that, I used to think organic canola oil was a decent compromise, but I've also recently learned that one aspect of the extraction process hydrogenates a significant proportion of canola oil, leading to the presence of dreaded trans fats. So now I'm not so sure. Grapeseed oil—generally made from the seeds of wine grapes—doesn't share those particular problems, but it can be pricier; it's also really hard to find as an organic product (which makes sense when you think

- Cornstarch (for thickening stews and curries)
- Dijon mustard
- Olive oil
- Polenta
- Soy sauce
- Steel cut oats (if you like oatmeal)
- Toasted sesame oil
- Tomato paste (look for this packaged in a tube; if you buy it in a can, it will go bad way before you can use it all up)

These are really great to have around if you think you'll use them, and they last forever:

- Barley (for when you get sick of eating your bean stews and fried tofu with rice)
- Boxed silken tofu**** (good as a component of egg substitute in baking and to puree into sauces)
- Boxed vegetable broth (I like the boxes better than cans; good for stronger flavor in soups and stews, though you can also always use water)
- Chipotles in adobo sauce (for extra easiness, puree a can of these in the food processor, stick the results in well-sealed container in the fridge, and use spoonfuls as needed)
- Dried fruit for snacking and putting in oatmeal

....

about how little wine is organic). But I am leaning toward thinking it's a better choice even if it's conventionally grown. However, I'm not entirely sure, and, furthermore, I haven't used grapeseed oil as extensively as I have canola, so I'm still listing canola in all my recipes.

**** Yes, soy is kinda controversial both health- and environmental footprint-wise. I still eat tofu and tempeh and recommend them; see my (brief) discussion of this in the introduction for more information.

- French green lentils (a.k.a. du Puy lentils or *lentilles du Puy*)
- Millet (also for when you get sick of eating your bean stews and tofu with rice; plus, try it for breakfast the way you would eat oatmeal)
- Nuts (whatever kind you like) for snacking and putting in breakfast porridges
- Nutritional yeast (for Debbie's Tempeh, page 69, and for adding a savory non-cheese cheesiness to anything you want)
- Peanut oil (Debbie insists that this is the secret to her tempeh, and it's also good for Asian-style stir-fries, but canola or grapeseed oil can be used instead)
- Quinoa (see what I said about millet, above)
- Sriracha (a Vietnamese condiment made from garlic and chiles; it's a nice little addition to things if you like spicy)
- Untoasted (a.k.a. light) sesame oil (good to have for the tofu recipe on page 64, but the deal here is the same as with peanut oil)
- Walnut oil (good for baking and, if you want some nuttiness in there, salad dressings)
- Whole wheat pasta (I may be unusual in not cooking much pasta; this may belong on your must-have list)

If you intend to bake, keep on hand:
- Applesauce (see the egg substitute point in "Tips and Techniques," page 39)
- Baking powder (aluminum-free)
- Baking soda
- Brown rice syrup and/or agave syrup
- Dried fruit, nuts, chocolate chips, and the like to put in your cookies

- Good cocoa powder and bittersweet chocolate
- Rolled oats if you like oatmeal cookies
- Sucanat (an unrefined sugar, the name comes from "sugar cane natural") or evaporated cane juice (you can use regular granulated and/or brown sugar, of course, but it's just not as good, both for flavor and health)
- Vanilla extract
- Whole wheat flour

You need to have these in your spice rack:

- Cayenne pepper (if you like to make anything spicy)
- Chili powder (a combo of chiles, cumin, oregano, garlic, and other spices, depending on the brand)
- Curry powder (each brand is different and some are hotter than others, so just find one you like)
- Dried rosemary (this is one of the few herbs that's just as good dried as it is fresh)
- Ground cinnamon (for baked goods and also oatmeal; some people like to put it in savory stuff like the chili- or Indian-style beans 'n' greens, so play around with that if it appeals to you)
- Ground coriander
- Ground cumin
- Kosher, sea, or mineral salt; I recommend avoiding regular table salt because it has added iodine and anti-clumping agents. But I also don't recommend spending real money on salt. There are a lot of fancy, spendy salts on the market, and though there are some textural differences that change the taste when you sprinkle them on top of food after it's done, for cooking they're pretty much all the same, so it doesn't really matter. However, the size of the crystals

determines how much salt fits in your measuring spoon. All of the recipes in this book give salt quantities for the average kosher or small sea salt texture. Kosher salt is widely and cheaply available at any supermarket, while nonfancy sea salt is available for under $2 a pound at any store with a good bulk section. If all you've got is regular table salt, reduce the amount in all of my recipes by one-third.

• Paprika (comes in hot and sweet varieties; I like hot but if you aren't so into spicy food, get the sweet)

• Red pepper flakes (again, if you like to cook things spicy)

• Turmeric

• Whole black peppercorns in a grinder (don't bother with pre-ground pepper; it tastes like dirt, literally)

You should think about having these in your spice rack:

• Cardamom pods

• Dried herbs such as oregano, thyme, dill, and bay leaves (these are very much fine in dried form and it may not be worth it to get them fresh, especially if you only need a little at a time)

• Fenugreek

• Garlic and onion powders (okay, these are kinda gross for most uses, but they're great in the tempeh recipe on page 69 and sprinkled on popcorn; you also may find other uses)

• Ground cardamom (sweeter than the whole pods; good for oatmeal and baked goods)

• Mustard seeds

• Powdered chiles in different varieties (this is not the same as chili powder; these are actually dried ground peppers, and if you run across them in your supermarket it's fun to experiment with them in my beans 'n' greens recipes or other bean stews)

- Whole cumin seeds

A FURTHER NOTE ON YOUR SPICE RACK: While fresh herbs are awesome and in most cases better than their dried counterparts, they're pricey and can be hard to find. Most generally available herbs are fine in their dried forms. The exceptions, in my opinion, are parsley, basil, and chives; you're better off using something else or skipping them altogether if you can't get those fresh. Also, powdered ginger is worse than useless unless you're baking something sweet where ginger is only a small element, like pumpkin pie. For a savory dish calling for dried ginger, just use fresh in a smaller quantity, and if you're looking at a gingerbread recipe that calls for powdered ginger, find a new recipe.

You need to have these at all times even though they will (eventually) go bad if you don't use them:
- Garlic
- Onions

You should try to have these around as much as possible even though they will (eventually) go bad if you don't use them:
- Ginger
- Lemons and/or limes
- Potatoes
- Sweet potatoes

You need to buy these frequently in small amounts because they go bad:
- Fresh fruit
- Fresh vegetables

- Tempeh and water-packed (not boxed) tofu

A NOTE ON STORAGE AND PERISHABILITY: When I say that something lasts forever, what I really mean is that it will generally last at least as long as it takes you to use it if you cook regularly (except canned beans and tomatoes—they really do last forever). Oils will eventually go rancid (and nut oils will do so faster than others), but if you store them away from strong heat and direct sunlight and you buy them in quantities appropriate to how often you use them, you'll be fine. Grains (and dried beans) can get kinda old and overly dry; you just may need some extra water and/or time to cook them. Spices and dried herbs do lose their flavor over time, but I'm not one of those people who insists that you have to replace everything in your spice rack every six months—that's just not practical. As with everything else, use your judgment.

tips and techniques
(a.k.a., why are you telling me to do it that way?)

SINCE I'M ENCOURAGING YOU TO EXPERIMENT AND USE the recipes in this book as templates, I want to explain a few things about how food works. Understanding a few basic techniques, quirky food facts, and applied-food-science concepts will equip you with more improvisational cooking skills and help you make sure your experiments go well.

- There are **three basic ways to cook vegetables**: sautéing, steaming, and blanching. (Okay, there are five, but roasting is fully covered on page 76 and boiling is really not a good idea for any veggie except corn, because you lose more flavor in the water and risk overcooking; one of the other methods is always better.) Each one is very simple. There's more info about sautéing in the recipes themselves, but here's the quick version: Heat some oil in a skillet or sauté pan over high heat (you might need to adjust to medium), toss veggies in, and stir occasionally until things are cooked. If it's burning or going too slow, you can cover the pan, and the water in your veggies will turn to steam, which will help the cooking process along. (I also recommend adding some garlic whenever you sauté vegetables.) To steam vegetables, put them in a steamer basket, set the basket in a saucepan or sauté pan (anywhere it fits) over a small amount of water (an inch or so usually does it), cover with a tight-fitting lid, and turn the heat on high. It can take as little as three minutes and as much as 10 or 20 depending on the vegetable and the size of the pieces. Just taste as you go. Blanching is actually a form of boiling, but it's more of a quick dunk in the water instead of full-on, stay-in-there-for-half-an-hour kind of thing. Blanching usually takes about half the time of steaming; delicate items like snow peas are usually done in a minute or less. It's easy to overcook things in boiling water, so keep a close eye and err on the side of pulling things out too early. (Also see the point about carryover cooking, below.)

- **Sautéing an onion—and/or some garlic, shallots, scallions, or leeks—is usually your first step to anything.** These vegetables, all members of the allium family, provide a great flavor base for so many dishes. Some alliums are milder than others (chives and leeks compared to garlic and onions, for example); some work well together (garlic with anything) and some just duplicate each other and so can be seen as interchangeable in a pinch or good candidates for swapping out in an experiment (say, leeks and scallions or shallots and red onions). Garlic cooks faster than other alliums, at least partly because you want to mince it more finely than anything else; it also tends to get bitter when it burns, so keep a close eye on it. If you're using more than one allium, always add the garlic last.

- **Sautéing spices in oil increases their flavor** (this is sometimes referred to as "blooming"). You'll notice that most of the recipes involve adding spices early on, when they can be sautéed in oil (usually along with an allium), and that's why. This works because it's volatile oils in the spices that give them their flavor. Thus, the most effective way to extract their flavor is also with oil, and heating brings out the flavor compounds further. It doesn't matter how much you understand or care about the process, though—the bottom line is that blooming in oil is important for actually getting the flavor from the spice into your food. Don't be tempted to skip this, even if it adds an extra step. And if you find that something you've made is underspiced, bloom whatever you're going to add in a small skillet before plopping it into the dish.

- **Don't skimp on oil and salt.** These two items have been unfairly demonized in U.S. food culture. Fat conveys flavor in your mouth and salt heightens it (i.e., it makes foods taste more like themselves), so if you don't use enough of either, your food just won't taste as good. Period, full stop. Of course, tastes vary about how much of either is too much or not enough, so you'll find the right balance for you through trial and error. But if you find yourself thinking, "All the flavors are here, but it's just not quite *enough*," consider the possibility that you have undersalted or not used enough oil.

- **Salt early** and taste for adjustments along the way. I find that salting only later on means the salt doesn't really penetrate the food well and you don't get as much flavor out of it. This is why I call for salting at the allium-sautéing stage. It seems to spread flavor throughout the dish. To avoid oversalting, be on the scant side at first and add a bit more with each new ingredient. That way you can taste along the way and see how you're doing. And of course each eater can always salt hir own portion at the table to top it off, but, like I said, I think salt sprinkled on top of food does less good.

- **Browning = flavor.** Browning happens when the sugars in your food get oxidized (with meat it's proteins, and called a Maillard reaction, but that's a different story); in addition to the pretty color, sugar oxidation releases chemical compounds that have the yummy, nutty, toasty-goodness flavors that make food taste good. So you want your food to get a little browned, especially onions and other alliums at the beginning of the sautéing process, tofu slabs on the griddle, and veggies in the roasting pan.

- **Deglazing** is the process by which tasty browned bits and accompanying flavor compounds get incorporated into your food while avoiding burning. You deglaze a pan by adding a little bit of liquid (water, broth, and wine all work well) when your food (in these recipes, usually alliums and spices) is dry and threatening to burn. The liquid will prevent burning and loosen the browned bits from the bottom of the pan. By the time you've stirred thoroughly and scraped the bottom of the pan with your spatula or wooden spoon, the liquid will be pretty much evaporated. You can then continue cooking the alliums and spices on their own if that's what you need to do. You can repeat this process as many times as you need to; each one means more flavor.

- The acids in tomatoes slow the cooking of onions, so you should **always wait until onions are fully cooked before adding any tomato products** such as tomato paste, crushed tomatoes, or fresh tomatoes.

- Speaking of which, **tomato paste is great for building richness of flavor,** so you may want to consider putting it in soups, stews, stir-fries, and the like even when you aren't planning for them to be particularly tomato-ey.

- **Dried herbs behave like spices** in that they benefit from long cooking and being sautéed in oil, but **fresh herbs lose their flavor with long cooking,** so you should add them toward the end of cooking time.

• **Pressing your tofu** is an extra step that's well worth it. Tofu has a lot of water in it, and getting that water out will a) make it easier for other flavors to get absorbed into the tofu and b) make your final dish not-watery. Pressing tofu is also incredibly simple. Take your block o' bean curd, slice it into slabs (half an inch to an inch thick is usually right), lay the slabs out on a clean dish towel (folded in half if it's big enough), cover with another clean dish towel, put a cookie sheet or large flat-bottomed pan on top, and put some heavy items on top of that. Cans of food or a full teakettle usually work well; just make sure everything's well balanced so it doesn't all fall over. Wait at least 20 minutes (this is often just the amount of time you need to prep your marinade or other food) or as long as an hour. P.S., paper towels will work if you don't have clean dishtowels, but you need a lot of them, so it's extra wasteful and not recommended.

• When you take something off the heat, it'll continue to get cooked by the heat remaining inside the food itself. This is called **carryover cooking**, and it applies to pretty much everything, though it only really matters when precision is important (like when you want your pasta or vegetables to be al dente; don't worry about it with soups and stews and the like). In these cases, err on the side of undercooking when you're pulling things off the heat. Carryover cooking is by far the most crucial when it comes to vegetables that are going to be served cold or at room temperature (such as in a salad). You'll need to bring their temperature down fast when they're done; otherwise, the residual heat can turn your beautiful, still-bright-and-a-little-crunchy green beans into a drab and mushy pile. The solution when it comes to vegetables cooked via a wet method (steaming or blanching) is a cold-water bath. Fill a big bowl with ice water and put your veggies into it as soon as they're out of the pot. In a pinch—say, if you don't have any ice—you can put them in a colander, run some cold water over them, and then put them in your freezer until they're no longer warm to the touch. For roasted or sautéed vegetables, carryover cooking isn't as big a deal because you haven't introduced any extra hot liquid into the inside of the vegetable, but if you're not going to eat them hot, you probably want to pull them out of the oven/off the burner a minute or two early and get them out of their hot pan to let the extra heat escape.

• The **easiest way to destem greens** is to grab the stem with both hands, like you're going to break the stem in half at the point where the leaf starts. Pull your hands in opposite directions, working the leaf off the stem with your fingers as you pull. Kale, collard, and mustard green stems should be discarded; they're too tough and woody to eat. Chard and beet green stems are yummy, though they take a bit longer to cook than the leaves, so it's generally a good idea to separate them anyway so you can add stems to your dish earlier than the leaves.

• The **easiest way to peel garlic** is to crush it with the side of your chef's knife. Lay the knife flat on top of a clove, hold the handle for stability while you put the palm of your other hand on top of the knife (being careful to stay away from the blade edge), and press down firmly. Once crushed, the paperlike peel will come right off the garlic.

• The **easiest way to wash a leek** thoroughly is to chop it before washing. Slice it in half lengthwise and then cut each half into half-inch pieces. Stick it all in a colander and run it under cold water.

• The **basic method of cooking any grain** is to boil lightly salted water (or broth, if you want to add some extra flavor) in a saucepan large enough to accommodate at least four times the uncooked volume of your grain, add the grain, cover tightly, turn heat to low, and simmer until the grain is tender and the water has been absorbed (you can always add more water if the liquid is gone but the grain is still too cruncy). Here are some liquid-to-grain proportions and approximate cooking times for common items: brown rice, two to one, 45 minutes; pearled barley, three to one, 45 minutes; hulled barley, three or four to one, an hour and a half; quinoa, two to one, 15 to 20 minutes; millet, three to one, 30 minutes; bulgur wheat, two to one, 20 minutes (though some bulgur is presteamed and should be prepared with the same method as couscous, described below); wheat berries, three to one, two hours. I recommend doing all this in a rice cooker, which is more forgiving and lets you throw water and grain together, push a button, and go do something else (see the equipment section, page 25). Grains generally expand to two to three times their uncooked volume during cooking. To make couscous, which is actually not a grain but a tiny little pasta, proportions of water to pasta are one to one, but instead of boiling the couscous, you add it to the boiling water, turn off the heat, cover it tightly, and let it sit for about five minutes or so until the liquid has been absorbed.

• **If you're making grains for a salad** or other cold dish, it's important to turn them out of the pan and into a large bowl that gives them plenty of space to let off steam; fluff them thoroughly with a fork to help that process along and separate the grains. A lot of cookbooks instruct you to do this for grains under all circumstances, but

I think mushiness or stickiness isn't really much of a danger unless the grains are bound for salad. Also, if your dressing is ready while the grains are cooling, pour a little bit over them. The heat left in the grains will help them absorb the flavors of the dressing better, and the dressing's oil will help the anti-stickiness cause.

• **If you're pan-frying** tofu or tempeh as described in the recipes for Ginger-Garlic-Sesame Tofu (page 64), Mustard-Rosemary Tofu (page 67), or Debbie's Tempeh (page 69) it's really easy to **add some veggies to your pan to complete the meal**, and extra marinade can flavor them as well if that sounds good to you. Spinach is the easiest. Once you've flipped the tofu slabs, smush some leaves around in the marinade and plop them on top of the tofu. The heat from the cooking tofu is enough to wilt the spinach. For longer-cooking greens, do the same thing, but plop them side by side with the protein, and do it a little earlier in the process so they have more time to cook. For harder veggies like broccoli, green beans, asparagus, or peas, cut them into bite-size pieces and start them at the same time or, in the case of broccoli, even before the tofu/tempeh. You also might need to sprinkle a little water over them to create some steam to help things along.

• Delicate greens such as **spinach** (and even other varieties if they are young and tender) **can be cooked by pouring boiling water on top** of them. It's not a technique worth using unless you're already pouring boiling water somewhere, but when you're making a pot of pasta it's an awesome shortcut to adding some veggies to your meal. Just put the greens in the colander and drain the pasta over them. If you don't have spinach, other veggies (broccoli, green beans, and the like) can be chopped and tossed into the pasta water a few minutes before draining (this is pretty much the only time I recommend boiling vegetables).

- **Some canned or frozen vegetables are useful and worth buying:** frozen corn, peas, and okra; canned tomatoes and corn. For anything else, you're generally better off finding something else you can use that's more available or in season.

- To turn a muffin, quick bread, or cookie recipe vegan, **an easy egg replacer** is (per egg) a well-blended combo of 1 tablespoon soft silken tofu, ½ tablespoon unsweetened applesauce, and 1 teaspoon prune puree. I buy applesauce in those little kids' lunch packages, which is a hideous amount of packaging, but it means that my applesauce doesn't go bad in between baking sprees. The prune puree is optional, but easy to make and keep around: Process equal parts prunes and water in a food processor until smooth; it keeps for quite a while in the fridge as long as it's in a container with minimal air. **To replace butter, use a neutral-tasting vegetable oil,** such as canola or grapeseed (see the footnote about these on page 32), or—if your item will taste good with any particular nut and you feel flush enough to spring for it, the oil of that nut. Quantity-wise, you want about 80 percent as much oil as the recipe calls for butter (butter has water in it, so unlike oil it's not 100 percent fat; you don't usually need to add extra liquid because the moisture in the tofu/applesauce egg replacer is generally enough).

- An easy way to make an unfancy dish like Lentils with Wine, page 59, or Greens Pie with Herbs and Lemon, page 101, into something a little more special is to **roll it into a package with phyllo.** You may have encountered phyllo in spinach pie or baklava—it's thin, flaky sheets of dough, and you can buy it frozen. I'm especially psyched about it now that there are whole-wheat and organic versions available. Your package will have some directions on it, but here's the basic method: Defrost your dough. Lay one piece on a cookie sheet or baking tray. Brush it with a thin layer of olive oil. Lay another sheet on top and do the same. Keep going until you have about ten sheets. Then spoon your filling onto the dough lengthwise, making a mound of filling along one side, leaving several inches of room at the edge and at each end. Roll the dough around the filling, folding the dough in at the sides as you go to fully enclose the filling. When it's all rolled up, roll it over seam-side down so its own weight keeps it closed. Then brush the whole thing with oil and bake it at 350°F for about a half an hour or so or until golden brown. A less pretty but easier and just as tasty option is to make phyllo-based pies in casserole pans by putting about five sheets of dough in the bottom (brush each with oil before adding more, as described above), laying the filling in there, and then topping with about ten more sheets.

recipes

chili-style beans 'n' greens

I started making bean stews with greens when I first began my veganesque whole-foods experiment. I'd been making vegetarian chilis for years, and often felt like they could use more vegetable action. Chard and kale hadn't really been a part of my life before, but it seemed like an appealing idea to toss them in the pot. I was right. Because it's pretty much the easiest thing in the world, this is probably the meal I make most frequently (though it might be tied for that status with roasted vegetables), with the other spice combinations (see the following two recipes) coming in close behind. You probably want to eat this over rice or some other grain.

🕐 Takes about 45 minutes. Serves four to six. It doubles well and also makes great leftovers, since the flavors continue to meld.

1 tablespoon olive oil (more if you like things richer, or if it just seems like a good idea)

1 large onion, chopped

1 teaspoon sea salt (or more to taste; also, see the note about salt textures and measurements in the pantry section)

4 cloves garlic, minced (or more if you love garlic)

3 tablespoons chili powder

1 tablespoon ground cumin

1 pinch cayenne (optional; or more if you want more heat)

1 tablespoon tomato paste

1 chipotle in adobo sauce or 1 generous teaspoon chipotle puree (optional; see notes)

1 large sweet potato, cut into bite-size chunks

1 15-ounce can diced tomatoes, including the juice (the
   ounceage is approximate here, but this is generally the
   standard can size)

1 bunch kale, destemmed and chopped (see note; discard
   stems)

1 15-ounce can black beans, drained and rinsed

1 15-ounce can kidney beans, drained and rinsed

2 cups water or veggie broth (I can't emphasize enough how
   approximate this is—you just want enough to barely
   cover all your stuff in the pot; you can always add more
   later, and if you add too much you can let it simmer longer, uncovered, until enough liquid boils off)

1. Heat the oil in a sauté pan or small stockpot (you want a four-
to six-quart capacity) over medium-high heat. Add the onion and
the salt and cook, stirring regularly, until onions are soft, about 10
minutes. It's not a bad thing if they get some brown on 'em.

2. Add the garlic and dry spices; turn the heat down to medium
so the spices don't scorch. Stir steadily and cook for another five
minutes or so. Keep an eye on it for burning or sticking–if the spice
mixture starts to stick to the bottom of the pot, add a tablespoon
or two of water and stir/scrape the bottom. You want to keep it all
from burning and keep the flavors you're generating in the food
and not stuck to the pot. (See the point about deglazing in "Tips
and Techniques," page 39, for information about this process.)

3. Add the tomato paste and chipotle. Cook for another minute
or two (or three).

4. Add the sweet potato and the diced tomatoes (with their

juice) and some water/broth to barely cover, if needed. Bring to a simmer and let it do its thing for 15 minutes or so. This might be a good point to taste and see if you need more salt. (See "Tips and Techniques," page 39, on salting.)

5. Add the beans and the kale along with more liquid if needed, and continue simmering until the beans are heated through and the kale is wilted and tender (about seven to 10 minutes, most likely). Taste, adjust seasoning, and serve—or keep simmering until you're ready.

notes

Chipotles in adobo are smoked jalapeños in a spicy sauce; they come in little cans in the Mexican aisle at the supermarket and bring a smoky, rich, tangy flavor and extra spiciness to whatever you put them in. The vinegar and spices in the adobo mean they keep forever in the fridge either whole or pureed in the food processor.

I like dino kale, a.k.a. lacinto kale, the best, 'cause I think it's less bitter, but use any variety you want. See "Tips and Techniques," page 39, for the easiest way to destem greens.

variations

• As the name indicates, any kind of greens will work here: spinach and chard, which are milder than kale; or collards, mustard greens, turnip greens, beet greens, or dandelion greens, all of which have pretty strong flavors, so you'll have to do some experimenting to see what works for you. In California, sweet potatoes and kale are readily available all year long, but in other regions this may be more of a fall and winter combination. Other good possibilities for winter are potatoes, winter squash, and carrots (add any of these as the same time as you would the sweet potatoes); in summer, try zucchini, corn, bell peppers, and/or green beans (add them later, more toward the kale point).

• For a classic vegetarian chili, use bell peppers as your only vegetable (add them where you would add the sweet potato; they don't take as long to cook, so you can shorten the time if you need to, but a classic chili has very thoroughly cooked peppers). Pressed and crumbled firm tofu or crumbled tempeh (make sure you get some without any added seaweed or other non-chili-compatible flavors) is also a nice addition.

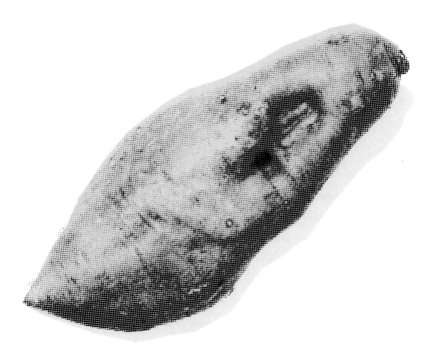

indian-style beans 'n' greens

This is probably the least authentic Indian meal ever, but the flavors are there and oh so tasty. Some of the spices may be hard to find—you can skip them if you need to; you'll lose some depth of flavor, but I promise it will still be good. This dish is especially nice on a cold and wet winter night.

⏱ Takes about 45 minutes. Serves four to six. It doubles well and also makes great leftovers, since the flavors continue to meld.

1 large onion, chopped

2 tablespoons olive oil (approximate, as always)

1 tablespoon mustard seeds

1 tablespoon whole cumin seeds

½ tablespoon fenugreek

6 cardamom pods

1 teaspoon sea salt (to taste, of course; also, see the note about salt textures and measurements in the pantry section)

1 tablespoon tomato paste

2 teaspoons ground cumin

1 teaspoon coriander

1 teaspoon turmeric

3 medium carrots, cut into rounds or chunks

3 medium potatoes, cut into (about) ½-inch cubes

1 bunch kale (dino, a.k.a. lacinto, preferred), destemmed and chopped

1 15-ounce can garbanzo beans (the ounceage is approximate here, but this is generally the standard can size)

3 cups water or broth (this is especially approximate, as you want to barely cover your other ingredients with liquid; you can adjust it to your desired texture by adding more water and/or by thickening it with cornstarch)

2 teaspoons cornstarch (for thickening; optional)

1. Heat the oil in a sauté pan or small stockpot (you want a four- to six-quart capacity) over high heat. When the oil is hot, turn the heat down a little; add the mustard seeds, cumin seeds, fenugreek, and cardamom pods and cook for about a minute (you'll know when to continue when the mustard seeds start popping).

2. Add the onion and cook, stirring regularly, until it starts to soften and become translucent, about five to seven minutes (you may need to turn the heat back up at first, because the cold onion will suck a lot of heat out of the pan).

3. Add the salt, ground cumin, coriander, turmeric, and tomato paste. Cook for another few minutes, stirring almost constantly. If things start to stick or burn, add a few tablespoons of liquid and stir especially vigorously, getting any browned bits off the bottom of the pan. (See the deglazing point in "Tips and Techniques," page 39, for information on why this is good.)

4. Add the carrots and potatoes. Stick a lid on there, lower the heat to the low side of medium, and let it all cook on its own for about 10 minutes. If it's dry or seems in danger of burning, add some more liquid. The quantity doesn't matter, since you're going to be adding more later anyway.

5. Add the kale and beans. Add enough liquid to barely cover everything. Bring to a simmer and cook, uncovered, for 15 to 20 minutes. It's ready to eat as soon as the carrots, potatoes, and kale are tender, but the longer it cooks the more the flavors will meld, so if you have time, just keep it going with the heat very low. Taste, and adjust the salt and other seasonings if necessary.

6. If desired, thicken with cornstarch: Spoon a half-cup or so of hot broth out into a bowl. Sprinkle the cornstarch into the hot broth while stirring; mix thoroughly and make sure there are no lumps. Add the mixture back into pot; stir, and then let it simmer for another few minutes (you'll see the texture of the liquid change).

variations

• You can use tofu instead of garbanzo beans (press water out of tofu as described on page 43 and cut it into cubes).

• Instead of kale, you can use chard, mustard greens, collards, or spinach. If you choose spinach, add it at the end, when you have about five minutes of cooking left. For everything else, the timing is the same.

• Instead of or along with the potatoes and carrots, you can use cauliflower (add it on the same timing as the kale; it can get mushy if it's cooked too long, though the flavor is good no matter what).

• These are just a few of the vegetable possibilities. The only really necessary items are the onion and the spices. As always, the possibilities are endless.

indian-style beans 'n' greens

italian-style beans 'n' greens

This one's a little lighter and less of a stew than the other beans 'n' greens combos.

⏱ Takes about a half an hour. Serves two to four and doubles easily. Keeps fine, though without the improvement of the other beans 'n' greens variations.

1 tablespoon olive oil (approximate)

1 medium leek, chopped

4 cloves garlic, minced (or less if you want)

1 scant teaspoon sea salt (see the note in the pantry section about salt textures and measurements)

1 teaspoon dried thyme, or 1 tablespoon fresh thyme

2 medium potatoes, cut into (about) ½-inch cubes

1 bunch kale (dino, a.k.a. lacinto, preferred), destemmed and chopped

¼ cup vegetable broth (see note)

1 15-ounce can white beans (a.k.a. cannelini; and yes, I am going to keep saying, once per recipe, that ounceage is approximate and I am simply referring to a standard can size)

1. Slice the leek in half lengthwise and then chop the halves into ¼-inch (or so) pieces. Put the chopped leek into a colander and rinse thoroughly. (This method is really the best way to make sure you·get all the dirt out from between the leek layers.)

2. Heat oil in a large sauté pan or small stockpot over medium heat. Add the leeks, garlic, and salt. Sauté for five minutes or so

(or however long it takes you to wash and cube the potatoes), until the leeks soften.

3. Add the potatoes and the thyme and let cook, covered, for about five minutes (or as long as it takes you to prep the kale).

4. Add the beans, kale, and broth. Stir, put the cover back on, turn the heat to low, and simmer until the potatoes and kale are tender.

note

Broth quantity is very approximate; how much moisture you need will depend on how much is already in your potatoes and greens. Also, you can use water instead, but because this is not a strongly spiced dish, broth really does increase its flavor significantly.

variations

• You can use onion (or any allium) instead of leeks.

• Parsley makes a good addition. Also, try swapping out the thyme for other herbs.

• Oddly enough for something called beans 'n' greens, this is just as good without the beans, though it becomes more of a side dish.

• It can also be turned into a soup with the addition of about two more cups of broth. You can leave it all as is, or puree it partially or fully with a stick blender.

lentils with wine

This is a streamlined version of a recipe in Deborah Madison's *Vegetarian Cooking for Everyone*. It's incredibly easy, yet also sophisticated in a way that impresses guests, especially when paired with sides like roasted root vegetables (see page 76), sautéed greens (see page 74), and/or pan-fried polenta (see page 71). Or toss some greens in with the lentils and eat it over rice all casual-like, by yourself.

🕐 Takes about 50 minutes, most of it simmering while you can go off and do something else. Serves four. Keeps well and doubles easily.

1 tablespoon olive oil

1 medium onion, chopped

1 teaspoon sea salt (to taste; also, see the note about salt textures and measurements in the pantry section)

1 tablespoon tomato paste

1 cup French green lentils (see note)

1 bay leaf

½ cup red wine

1½ cups water

1 tablespoon dijon mustard

1 teaspoon red wine vinegar

pepper to taste

1. Heat the olive oil over high heat in a sauté pan or large saucepan. Add the onion and salt and cook until the onion is soft, about 10 minutes. A little browning is good, but you don't want to burn anything, so you may need to adjust the heat downward.

2. Add the tomato paste and cook for another minute or two. If the pan is dry or if things seem in danger of burning, add a splash of the wine (see "Tips and Techniques," page 39, on deglazing, to see why this is a good thing to do). Keep cooking until the onion is well and truly cooked.

3. Add the lentils, the bay leaf, the rest of the wine, and the water. Cover, bring to a simmer, lower the heat, and let it do its thing for 35 minutes.

4. Stir in the dijon and the vinegar. Taste the lentils and see if they're done. If they're not soft enough, add a bit more water and keep simmering until they are done.

note

Unlike most other recipes, this is one where a main ingredient substitution won't work. French green lentils, which are also known as du Puy lentils or *lentilles du Puy* if you're really getting schmancy, aren't actually green—they're more brown with a green tinge—but they are the only ones that will hold their shape well enough to work in this dish. Others will fall apart and become soupy.

variations

• Try adding different herbs, such as rosemary, mint, or parsley. Dried herbs go in with the bay leaf, fresh after the lentils have been simmering for 30 minutes (see the pantry section, page 31, for tips on which herbs work well dried).

• Try adding different vegetables like carrots and celery (chop them relatively small and add them along with the tomato paste), or fruits like apples (chopped into small chunks) or currants (add these after the lentils have been simmering for about 20 minutes).

japanese-style tofu curry

This is classic comfort food that I discovered through my ex-husband. We used to buy these packages of curry mix that were totally delectable. Years later, when I realized how much MSG and god knows what else was in the mix, I wondered if I could duplicate the savory goodness. It turned out to be shockingly easy. Serve over rice.

⏱ Takes about 50 minutes. Serves four to six; keeps and doubles well.

> 1 tablespoon olive oil
>
> 1 large onion, chopped
>
> 1 teaspoon sea salt (start with this and add more later if
>   needed; be especially careful if you're using broth, since
>   it has its own salt)
>
> 3 cloves garlic, minced (or more or less, to taste)
>
> 3 tablespoons curry powder
>
> 4 carrots cut into rounds or chunks
>
> 4 ribs celery, chopped into pieces a little smaller than your
>   carrot pieces, preferably with some leaves included
>
> 4 medium potatoes, cut into ½-inch cubes
>
> 1 package firm or extra-firm tofu, pressed as described on
>   page 43 and cut into ¾-inch cubes (most packages are
>   12 ounces, but some are more and that's fine)
>
> 2 teaspoons cornstarch
>
> 4 cups broth or water

(cont.)

1 cup frozen peas (this is the only time I'll specifically tell you to use anything frozen, but fresh shelling peas should be enjoyed raw as a snack; it's a waste to cook them)

1. Heat the oil over high heat in a pot with at least a four- to six-quart capacity. Add the onion and salt and cook for about five minutes, stirring pretty often. Turn the heat down to medium; add the garlic and cook another minute or two, continuing to stir regularly. Add the curry powder and keep cooking and stirring until the onions are translucent. If the curry powder is burning or sticking to the bottom of the pan, add a bit of liquid (see the talk of deglazing on page 42). You can also turn the heat down; in this dish, you don't want to get too much brown on your onions.

2. Add the carrots, celery, potatoes, and a half-cup or so of liquid. Put a lid on the pot; turn the heat down if it's really sizzling in there. Cook for about 10 minutes, stirring every few minutes and adjusting the heat so it's not burning.

3. Add tofu and the rest of the liquid. Simmer, still covered, for about 20 minutes.

4. Thicken with cornstarch: Spoon a half-cup or so of hot broth out into a bowl. Sprinkle the cornstarch over the hot broth while stirring; mix thoroughly, making sure there are no lumps. Add the mixture back into pot and stir.

5. Add the peas and stir; simmer until broth has thickened and peas are hot through. Taste and adjust salt if needed.

japanese-style tofu curry

variations

• Like everything else, you can use whatever vegetables you want in here and/or use beans (especially garbanzos) instead of tofu. But tofu with onions, carrots, celery, potatoes, and peas is a traditional combination (my ex would insist that we had to make something else if any one of these ingredients was missing), so I'm just going to leave it all up to your imagination.

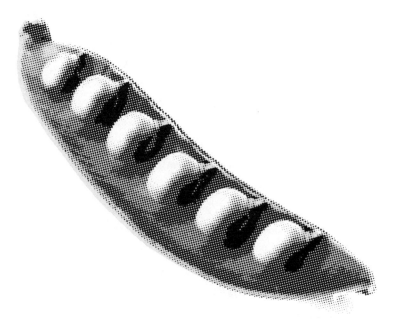

ginger-garlic-sesame tofu with spinach

The first time I used this marinade, I made little kebabs that I served at a party at my house. I didn't really think many people were going to want tofu on a stick in that setting, but they disappeared immediately and everyone thought I was some kind of genius. As much as I would love to take all the credit, it really should go to Deborah Madison, since it's her marinade. The idea of making it a complete meal by adding veggies right there to the tofu pan is all mine, though. I eat this over rice.

⏱ Takes about 20 minutes of active time and at least 20 minutes (but as much as you can give it) of marinating time. Serves between one and four at a time (you can fry up as much tofu as you want and leave whatever's left sitting in the marinade for up to a week). Doubles easily as long as you have enough space to spread your tofu in a single layer in the marinade.

1 package firm or extra-firm tofu (usually between 12 and 16 ounces; any size will do as long as it will feed the number of people you want to feed)

6 cloves garlic, minced (see notes)

1 2-inch piece of ginger, grated (see notes)

2 tablespoons light (a.k.a. untoasted) sesame oil (you can use peanut or a more neutral-tasting oil like canola [see the footnote about canola on page 32] instead if you don't want to invest in this)

1 tablespoon toasted sesame oil

3 tablespoons soy sauce

1 pinch red pepper flakes (optional, or more to taste)

1 teaspoon sucanat, honey, or other natural sweetener (the
   amount is very flexible; I often leave this out altogether,
   but some people like it with as much as a tablespoon of
   sweetener)

1 bunch spinach, washed and chopped, or ½ pound baby
   spinach leaves (or less, depending on how many people
   you're serving; you want about two big handfuls per person, since spinach cooks down so much)

1. Press your tofu as described on page 43.

2. Mix all the other ingredients (except spinach) together in a wide, shallow bowl or pie plate (basically, anything where you can spread the tofu slabs out in a single layer). Add the pressed tofu slabs, making sure to coat both sides with the marinade. Let sit, covered and refrigerated if it's going to be longer than about an hour, for at least 20 minutes and up to a week (overnight is ideal).

3. Heat a griddle pan or a skillet over high heat. No need to add oil, because the marinade has plenty.

4. Put your slabs in the pan and don't touch 'em for five minutes. Then start checking to see if they're brown on the bottom. When they are, flip 'em over.

5. Once you've flipped the tofu, smush the spinach around in the remaining marinade and plop the leaves on top of the slabs. The heat from the cooking tofu is enough to wilt the spinach. Let it all sit there frying until the tofu is brown on the second side.

notes

Six cloves of garlic generally adds up to about two tablespoons, but not only do amounts depend on your personal taste, but marinades are especially approximate because the herbs and spices aren't actually ending up in the finished dish.

To grate the ginger, use the small holes of a box grater or, if you use ginger a lot, get yourself a ginger grater, which is a porcelain or ceramic thing with dull teeth that tear the root apart. You could also mince it, but its stringiness makes that kinda difficult. You can peel it or not–since it's for a marinade and not going directly into the final product, it doesn't matter so much (especially if you have a ginger grater, since it will shred the meat of the root and leave the peel in your hand). As far as quantity goes, the idea is to have generally equal amounts of ginger and garlic, but, as always, feel free to adjust to your liking.

variations

• Try vegetables other than spinach; you can use pretty much anything you want. I tend to go for green things only: other greens, green beans, snow or snap peas, asparagus, broccoli. For longer-cooking greens than spinach, follow the directions above, but plop the leaves side by side with the tofu, directly on the pan, and do it more toward the beginning of cooking. For harder veggies like broccoli, green beans, asparagus, or peas, cut them into bite-size pieces and start them at the same time or even (in the case of broccoli) before the tofu. You might need to sprinkle a little water over them to create some steam to help things along.

• The fried tofu slabs also make a great sandwich on whole-grain toast with raw or wilted spinach, or a bitter salad green like arugula.

• The same method is used for Mustard-Rosemary Tofu on the next page.

mustard-rosemary tofu
with the vegetable of your choice

I've always thought of this marinade as my mother's—she used to make leg of lamb prepared this way when I was growing up—but when I told her I was using it for tofu and putting it in the book, she told me that it's actually an old Julia Child recipe. I still think of it as my mom's, though. Serve with roasted potatoes, couscous, barley, or rice.

⏰ Takes about 20 minutes of active time and at least 20 minutes (but as much as you can give it) of marinating time. Serves between one and four at a time (you can fry up as much tofu as you want and leave whatever's left sitting in the marinade for up to four or five days). Doubles easily as long as you have enough space to spread your tofu in a single layer in the marinade.

1 package firm or extra-firm tofu (usually between 12 and 16 ounces; any size will do as long as it will feed the number of people you want to feed)

2 tablespoons olive oil

4 tablespoons dijon mustard

2 tablespoons soy sauce

1 clove garlic, minced or crushed (or add another for extra garlic flavor)

1 generous teaspoon dried rosemary or 1 tablespoon fresh rosemary

the vegetable of your choice in the amount of your choice (I like green beans best for this dish)

1. Press your tofu as described on page 43.

2. Crush the rosemary with your fingers (if dried) or remove the leaves from the woody stems and chop them (if fresh). Mix all ingredients (except the tofu and your vegetable) together in a shallow dish. Add the tofu slabs, making sure to coat both sides with marinade. Let sit, covered and refrigerated if it's going to be longer than about an hour, for at least 20 minutes and up to four or five days (at least five hours or so is ideal).

3. Follow the method for Ginger-Garlic-Sesame Tofu with Spinach, page 64, starting with step 3 and following whatever the variation instructions are for the vegetable of your choice.

variations

- The fried tofu slabs make a great sandwich on whole-grain toast with raw or wilted spinach (or any kind of lettuce) and, in summer, sliced tomatoes.

debbie's tempeh

This recipe is from my friend who really got me started along the whole-foods, animal-products-aware path. I never considered cooking tempeh at home before she made it for me. It's great with roasted vegetables or sautéed spinach (or other greens), green beans, or broccoli (see "Tips and Techniques," page 39). You also might want some rice.

⏱ Takes about 15 minutes. Serves two to four, depending on what else you make with it. Doubles well, but I can't say that leftover tempeh appeals to me at all.

1 package tempeh (these are usually 10 ounces or so)

1 teaspoon garlic powder

1 teaspoon onion powder

1 teaspoon nutritional yeast

1 tablespoon soy sauce

peanut oil (enough to thinly coat the bottom of your pan; see note)

1. Cut tempeh into one-inch cubes and combine with all other ingredients (except oil) in a small bowl. Toss it all around so that the spices coat the tempeh fully.

2. Heat the oil in a skillet over medium-high heat and add the tempeh in a single layer. Fry it up and turn the pieces when they get browned, trying to hit all sides of all cubes.

3. That's it, you're done!

(cont.)

note

Debbie insists that peanut oil is the magic ingredient here, though I like it with any oil as long as it's cooked long and hot enough to get crispy, so if you're not going to use peanut oil for anything else and you're not sure how much tempeh you're going to be frying, you can start with canola (see the footnote about canola on page 32) or olive.

variations

• The principle here is using some liquid (soy sauce, broth, oil, etc.) to get some flavors to adhere to the tempeh. You can use whatever flavors you want: Try cumin and coriander. Try curry powder. Try chili powder. Just remember, if your flavor combination doesn't call for soy sauce, don't forget to add a healthy amount of salt to the mix.

• Also, check out Lisa P.'s Crack Spice Rub, page 89.

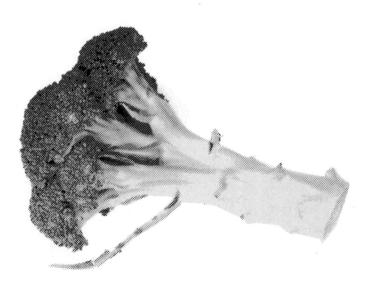

debbie's tempeh

spring vegetable sauté over polenta

This is one of those elegant items that impresses people and is so simple it's almost embarrassing. I started making it as part of my gluten-free repertoire, but it was so good I put it in regular rotation.

⏱ Takes about 45 minutes, including letting the polenta cool as needed. Serves four. Doubles well and keeps either well (if you like cold vegetables, which I do) or not so well (they'll get overcooked in the reheating). The polenta keeps great, though—you can make extra and fry it up later.

1 cup polenta

3 cups water

1½ teaspoons sea salt, some for the polenta and some for the sauté (see the note about salt textures and measurements in the pantry section)

1 large leek (or one of the following: a small bunch spring onions, a small bunch scallions, five cloves or more garlic, a large clump of shallots, or a medium onion)

1 tablespoon olive oil (or more if desired)

1½ pounds of one of the following: asparagus, woody parts of stems removed and the rest cut into 2-inch pieces; snap peas, stems and strings removed; spinach, chopped; zucchini, sliced into rounds or half-rounds depending on size; or some combination of any of these

¼ cup sun-dried tomatoes, softened in a small amount of hot water

1. First, make the polenta. Bring the water to a boil in a small saucepan with ½ teaspoon of the salt. While stirring, add the polenta slowly. Lower the heat so the mixture is lightly simmering. Cook, stirring constantly (or almost constantly) until the water has been absorbed/has evaporated and the polenta is thick enough so that your spoon can almost stand up on its own. Rub a 9-inch square baking pan with olive oil and pour the polenta into it to firm up. (If you don't have a 9-inch square, any baking pan, a pie plate, or anything with sides will work.) Set aside to cool and become firm.

2. In a large skillet or sauté pan, sauté your leek or other allium in the olive oil with the remaining 1 teaspoon of salt over medium heat until softened/translucent.

3. Add your prepared vegetables. If you're using more than one kind, you'll need to let some cook before adding the others (see note for more information). Stir, cover, turn heat to low, and cook for a minute or so while you chop the softened dried tomatoes.

4. Add the tomatoes to the veggies along with some of the soaking water (how much depends on what kind of veggies you're using: asparagus can take more water, peas slightly less, and spinach or zucchini very little). Keep the pan covered and stir/check for doneness every couple minutes (see note). The veggies should be bright and tender.

5. While the veggies cook, heat a small skillet or griddle over high heat and pour in enough olive oil to make a thin film on the pan. Cut the cooled polenta into squares (it will have firmed up quite a bit; if it hasn't, stick it in the freezer to cool faster) and fry them, flipping over when lightly browned and crispy on the bottom.

6. If the veggies finish before the polenta, just turn off their heat and keep them covered.

7. When everything's done, put the polenta squares on plates (two or three per person depending on how big you cut them and how hungry people are) and spoon veggies on top.

note

If you're using a combination of vegetables, you'll want to add some first and others later depending on how fast they cook. Asparagus takes about 10 minutes, snap peas and zucchini about seven, and spinach five or less.

variations

• You can leave out the sun-dried tomatoes, but not only do they provide a nice tang, your food will look a lot more boring without the color contrast they provide.

• If you've got fresh herbs, they'd be a great addition, especially parsley or basil. Add about a tablespoon, chopped, along with the veggies, and stir in another tablespoon right at the end, after you've turned the heat off.

• This is always good with parmesan cheese sprinkled on top, but it's totally optional.

• This can also be served over pasta, quinoa, barley, or rice.

• And perhaps it's too obvious to need stating, but try it in different seasons with different seasonal vegetables.

simple garlicky greens

There's not much more I can say about this than the title. It's a great side dish for almost anything, or even a light meal when paired with some kind of grain and a hunk of cheese or some nuts. Or put it on whole-grain toast for a quick snack. Mmmm, garlic.

⏱ Takes about five to 15 minutes. Serves one to six or more, depending on quantities and uses. Keeps and increases well.

a pound or 2 any kind of green (spinach, which will cook down more than the others, so just know that when you make decisions about quantity; chard; kale; collards; mustard, turnip, or beet greens; watercress; pea sprouts, if you are lucky enough to shop somewhere that has them; broccolini, ditto)

many cloves of garlic (one if you're not a garlic fiend, as many as seven or more if you are)

1 tablespoon or so olive oil

salt and pepper to taste

1. Mince the garlic and throw it in a sauté pan over medium heat with the oil and some salt. Cook for a couple minutes, until the garlic is soft and fragrant. Turn down the heat if it starts to brown; garlic burns easily and, unlike other alliums, browning can make it bitter.

2. Wash, destem (if necessary), and chop your greens (watercress and pea sprouts should be left whole) and toss them into the pan.

3. Stir and cover; let cook until greens are at their desired tenderness (timing will depend on the kind of greens: from three minutes for spinach to 12 minutes for kale; just keep checking and stirring and adjusting the heat).

4. Grind some pepper over it and you're done.

variations

• Add a teaspoon or so of balsamic vinegar at the very end (best on spinach, kale, and chard).

• Add a teaspoon (more if you think it needs it after tasting) of toasted sesame oil at the very end (good on everything). You could also take the Asian-style thing further here by replacing the olive oil with untoasted sesame oil, peanut oil, or canola oil (see the footnote about canola on page 32) and replacing the salt with soy sauce.

• Add a small handful of pine nuts along with the garlic, and a small handful currants or raisins (plumped in some hot water first if they are hard) at the very end (best on spinach, kale, and chard).

• I really do think garlic is best here, but if you've somehow run out and you really want some sautéed veggies, forage in your kitchen for any of the other alliums.

• You can also cook green beans, asparagus, broccoli, snow peas, or snap peas this way.

roasted vegetables

I got into roasting after reading Barbara Kafka's most excellent (if very meat-oriented) *Roasting: A Simple Art*; her advice and recipes laid the foundation for my veggie-roasting explorations. I am a vegetable-roasting fiend. I eat them just about every day in winter and almost once a week even in summer, as long as it's not *too* too hot out. My favorites are Brussels sprouts and sweet potatoes, with beets, cauliflower, and romanesco (a broccoli-cauliflower hybrid) coming in close behind.

There are a lot of variables that go into roasting vegetables, all of which will affect your results, so it's more important to understand how it all works than to have a set of instructions you can follow strictly (as you can see by the way I have listed the ingredients below). So, be warned, the notes are verbose; when I've tried to explain roasting methods simply and concisely to my friends ("Cut things into bite-size pieces, smush them around on a baking sheet with some salt and olive oil, and put them in a very hot oven for 20 or so minutes, stirring partway through"), they complain that their vegetables don't come out as well as mine. So, like with all my other recipes, you should do things your own way. But do take the time to read this whole thing. Really.

⏱ Takes about half an hour. Serves as many people as you have space on your trays to roast vegetables for. I love roasted veggie leftovers, but you might not.

some vegetables (for instance, asparagus, beets, broccoli, Brussels sprouts, carrots, cauliflower, parsnips, potatoes,

rutabagas, romanesco, sweet potatoes, turnips, winter
squash)

some olive oil (for things that can be cut into smooth-sided
cubes, it's 1 to 1½ tablespoons per pound of veggies; for
things with florets or lots of nooks and crannies [broccoli
and the like], you'll want more in the neighborhood of
2½ tablespoons per pound)

salt to taste (I recommend a scant half teaspoon [⅜, really]
of sea salt per pound of veggies; see the note about salt
textures and measurements in the pantry section)

pepper to taste (optional)

1. Read all the notes below. Roasting vegetables is an art, not a science, and there's a lot of flexibility in it. You'll get better results by understanding all the variables than by following any instructions to the letter.

2. Preheat your oven to 500°F. Yes, really: 500°F.

3. Cut your vegetables into the desired size pieces. The notes have more information, but in general, this means cubes of about a ½ inch by 1 inch by ¾ inch for things that can be cubed (potatoes, sweet potatoes, beets, etc.); for things with florets (broccoli and cauliflower), it means pieces about 2 inches long, 1 inch across (or ½ inch across as a stem), and ½ wide the other way (cut floretless stems into pieces just a bit bigger than the cubes described above). For other shapes, like carrots and parsnips, it means pieces 1 inch long for smaller ones and ½ inch long for wider ones. Average-size Brussels sprouts should be cut in half, really large ones should be quartered, and really small ones should be left whole. Asparagus should be roasted whole.

4. Put the veggie pieces on your baking sheet; drizzle the oil over 'em and toss the salt on top. Get your hands in there and rub it all together, making sure all the pieces are well coated on all sides/ in all nooks and crannies. The amounts listed above are a good guideline, but pay more attention to the look and feel of the veggies than any numbers. They should be slick and shiny all over–not dry, but not with oil pooling underneath them, either.

5. When your oven is ready (make sure it really is at 500°F; I usually wait another five minutes after my oven makes its "preheating is finished" sound), put your pan in there and set a timer for 12 minutes. When time is up, stir thoroughly to get different veggie surfaces exposed to the pan (see the notes!). Then put the pan back in the oven for another six or seven minutes (five if things seem like they're going fast and eight if they're going slow).

6. When time is up again, taste a piece (or poke it with a fork; it should yield pretty easily) to make sure it's done. If it's too crunchy, give your veggies another minute or two; keep doing that until they're ready. Grind pepper on top if you want, and eat! Yum.

notes (a.k.a. my novellini on the art of roasting vegetables)

First of all, you should know that when I roast, my goal is to get the veggies fully cooked through with a nice dark brown crust on the surface; I also like things a little rustic and with some variation in texture. These preferences determine how I do things and inform my determination of temperature, chopping, and timing. If you want things to be different, you'll want to make adjustments based on the information in these here notes.

The big variables These are the pan, the oven temperature, the size and shape of the vegetables, how crowded they are in the pan, and how long you cook them for. (Smaller variables–the amount of oil, the placement of individual pieces on the pan, placement of your oven racks, and how thoroughly you stir your veggies partway through cooking–will be covered later). All these variables interact with each other, and everyone's ovens and pans behave differently, so no matter what I tell you, you're going to have to do some experimenting to figure out what works best (and what you like, of course).

I know this all sounds complicated, but it's really not. The great thing about all the variables is that you can use them and their interactions to your advantage (you can get away with less oil in a more crowded pan, for instance, but you'll also get less browning because the veggies will steam each other a little bit; you can correct things midway through by adding oil, moving things around in the oven or on the pan, etc.). Also, like with anything else, when you roast vegetables more than a few times, you'll start to get a feel for how it all works.

The first thing you need is a good, solid, relatively heavy (to resist warping) metal pan. Glass or ceramic doesn't hold heat the same way as metal; don't ask me to explain it, just believe me when I tell you it won't brown your food right. The ideal thing to use is a jelly-roll pan (basically a cookie sheet with inch-high sides) or a half-sheet pan (a restaurant-supply-store word for a pan that's just like a jelly-roll pan and is, unlike many things sold at restaurant supply stores, the right size for a regular home oven). There are two reasons why a jelly-roll pan is ideal. The first is that you can get a lot of stuff on there without worrying that your veggies will fall off when you're moving the pan around, as they will if you use a plain ol' flat cookie sheet. The second is that you need the sides of your pan to be very low, because if they're any higher than an inch, they'll trap the moisture coming off the food and your stuff will steam rather than roast, leading to soft, not-browned, not-nearly-as-tasty veggies. The browning-versus-steaming thing is clearly more important, so if your choice is a brownie or loaf pan versus a cookie sheet, go with the flat sheet and be extra careful not to knock any pieces off when you stir. Also, nonstick surfaces are tempting, but don't do it. They interfere with browning, plus they can release toxic fumes at high temperatures.

Dark pans will generally absorb more heat and thus produce more intense browning. Light and/or shiny ones reflect instead of absorb. You can go with either; it's just good to know that there's a difference and what the difference can mean. If you're going to be roasting a lot, you'll want to season your pan well (basically, use it only for veggie roasting or other things that involve oil and not a lot of liquid, and don't wash it very often—just wipe it off with a paper towel or dishcloth between uses; you also might want to coat it with oil and roast it empty a few times when you first get it). I have two pans that I use only for roasting veggies; one's a jelly-roll pan and one's a pizza pan, so it has no sides, but once I started using it, it got seasoned so I just kept using it.

Next topic: oven temperature. To get the kind of browning I think is ideal, you really need to get it up to 500°F. If you have an oven thermometer, use it. If you don't, try to get one. I know my attitude about kitchen equipment is make-do thriftiness, but if you don't know how hot your oven is, it's going to stand in your way with roasted veggies (and baked goods, but that's another cookbook). Also, don't trust your oven to be fully heated when whatever built-in thermostat says it is. I always wait a few minutes after my oven thinks the preheating is done, 'cause in my experience that's just what needs to happen for it to really be at 500°F. If you want things less browned or you want to make sure you have no burned bits (though I think some burned bits are a risk well worth taking), then lower the temperature to 400°F and cook things longer.

On chopping the vegetables: Size and shape are what determines how long it takes something to get cooked, because they affect the amount of surface area exposed to the hot pan and the hot air, and the ratio of surface area to veggie bulk. To get even cooking—to have all your vegetables be done at the same time—you need to cut things into even pieces. However, I'm far from a chopping authoritarian. Not only do I dislike worrying about the exact measurements of my sweet potato chunks, but when eating I enjoy the slight texture differences that come from having pieces of veggies of slightly different sizes cooked for the same amount of time: some get crispier and more browned than others, some are chewier than others; it's just better. Plus, I like cooking different veggies on the same pan. So I've given some rough guidelines below about size and shape (and they go along with what I've said about time), but they're far from set in stone—as with anything, you should do it the way you like it best. If you don't want variations in texture, then cut things to uniform sizes and don't mix different vegetables together. If you want something done faster, cut the pieces smaller (with the caveat that smaller pieces will brown and burn faster, too, so you'll need to keep a close eye on everything and also have a carbon tolerance—or turn down the heat).

The next important thing is how full your pan is. For good browning, your vegetable pieces must be in a single layer with adequate space in between them. When they don't have about ¼ inch of space each, the result is similar to a pan with too-high sides: the moisture the veggies are giving off can't evaporate fast enough and they steam each other. So you don't want to crowd the pan too much. Some tiny spaces or even touching is okay (obviously you don't have to stand over the pan for half an hour arranging a halo of space around each veggie chunk–that's a little... much), but any stacking, or a wall-to-wall veggie carpet, will give you mushy, pale veggies. This can also be used to help you out if you've miscalculated something and, when you open the oven to stir, you see that browning is happening faster than actual cooking–that is, if your veggies are getting good color, or too much color, but they still seem on the raw side. When that happens, you can crowd them together in the middle of the pan, or even mound them up a bit, to make them cook through faster and keep from burning. If you have too much stuff for one sheet, use two (just make sure to also switch the rack positions when you take your veggies out to stir them).

Length of cooking time is also, obviously, very important. As noted in the instructions, I think that 17 to 20 minutes is right for most situations. But this is the variable most affected by the pan and the oven (not just the temperature, but the hot spots and cooler spots that every oven has). It's also the easiest to adjust on the fly–you just pull your trays out of the oven early or leave them in longer. In the end, you just have to keep checking to tell–by poking and tasting–when things are done.

roasted vegetables

The small variables To elaborate on the guidelines I've given in the ingredients list about how much oil to use: Either extreme is bad—not enough oil and your veggies will dry out and burn rather than brown; too much and they'll be greasy and the taste of oil can overwhelm the other flavors—but there's a lot of room in the middle there that's totally fine, and what's best is largely a matter of taste. Also, note that more oil generally means faster cooking. Floretted or otherwise irregular shapes take more oil, 'cause they have more surface area to coat than flat or smooth veggies.

You always want to stir your veggies partway through cooking to expose different surfaces to the hot pan (the face-up parts will brown from the heat, too, but not as nicely or flavorfully as the ones that touch metal). I think two-thirds of the way through is ideal; I stir after 12 minutes. While it would be great to be as thorough as possible and flip each vegetable piece individually, it just doesn't make sense to take the time to do that, so I take a spatula and turn swaths of the pan over and then redistribute the pieces. The one exception is Brussels sprouts. I do take the time with these, partly because I feel it makes a big difference, and partly because their shape makes it easy. I always start my sprouts with their cut sides down, and turn them individually with my hands to have their cut sides up. Yes, I am that much of a roasted sprouts geek. Okay then, moving on.

Another small variable is the placement of the pieces on the pan. Pieces toward the edge of the pan get browned faster, so you want to keep your smaller pieces toward the center to keep them from burning.

If you've got more than one pan to go in the oven at once, you also want to think about which pan to put where. I tend to put floretted items, brussels sprouts, and other non-square things on the bottom first (closer to the heat source), for the longer time. Then I switch racks after stirring. Regardless of what placement choices you make, though, if you have more than one pan, you always want to switch racks after stirring.

Parting thoughts Broccoli can be cut into bigger pieces than cauliflower because the florets tend to be more open/less compact, and so there's more surface area for the heat to come into contact with. With any floretted veggie, there are gonna be small pieces in there that get burnt. Think of them as providing extra texture and flavor. You can mix different kinds of vegetables together on one pan, but I find it useful to keep them confined to their own regions of the pan, in case one veggie is cooking faster than another and you want to do some mounding or whatever. Also, with beets, the juice will stain the other veggies, which isn't the end of the world, but I like to avoid it (also for that reason, I chop my beets last and also salt/oil/mush them last).

While anything can be roasted, I'm not crazy about it for zucchini and other summer squash (too watery), green beans (doesn't benefit their flavor), or peas of any kind (ditto). I also don't ever roast bell peppers except when they're an ingredient in another recipe, and in that case I always just do it over the burner. But you may feel differently, so I encourage you to play around with different veggies.

variations

• You may want to add herbs and spices to your roasted vegetables; for dried herbs, add them when you stir partway through, and consider lowering the heat afterwards. For fresh herbs, stir them in for the last minute or so of cooking. For spices, smush them on with the oil and salt and lower the heat to 450°F and/or keep a close eye out for burning and be prepared to lower the heat further. Some good combinations are potatoes and rosemary, sweet potatoes and cumin or chili powder, carrots and dill (if you like dill, which frankly I don't), and garlic with everything (treat whole, unpeeled cloves like just another veggie chunk, coating them with oil and roasting them for about 20 minutes total). Also see Lisa P.'s Crack Spice Rub, page 89, for more ideas.

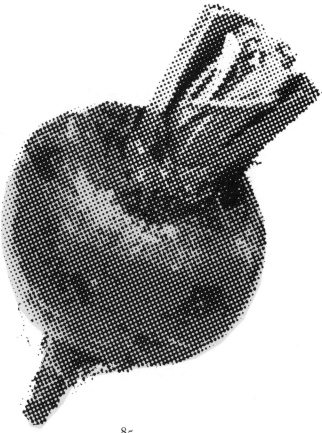

mustard-cilantro sauce

This is great as a dip, plus you can put it over pasta or rice with wilted greens or any blanched veggies for a quick meal (see "Tips and Techniques," page 39, and "Nonrecipe Recipes," page 113). Not to be a broken record or anything, but this is also based on a recipe from Deborah Madison.

🕐 Takes about 10 minutes. How many people it serves really depends on how you're using it. It'll keep in the fridge for a couple weeks, so it can just be good to make and have around.

1 12-ounce box soft silken tofu

2 teaspoons rice vinegar or lime juice

2 teaspoons sucanat or other sweetener

½ cup dijon mustard

salt to taste

2 small handfuls cilantro, chopped

1. Put everything except the cilantro in the bowl of a food processor fitted with the s-shaped metal blade. Process until smooth.

2. Stir in cilantro.

3. Taste and adjust seasonings if necessary.

note

If you don't have a food processor, you can mix this up with a stick blender or a hand mixer, or even with a wooden spoon if you're prepared to put in some serious work, but the texture won't be as smooth.

peanut sauce

This is basically the same idea as the last recipe: great as a dip or over pasta or rice with wilted greens or any blanched veggies.

🕐 Takes about 10 minutes. How many people it serves really depends on how you're using it. It'll keep in the fridge for a couple weeks, so it can just be good to make and have around.

1 12-ounce box soft silken tofu

¼ cup toasted sesame oil

½ cup tahini or unsweetened peanut butter (or a combination of the two adding up to ½ cup)

⅓ cup soy sauce or more to taste

2 tablespoons rice vinegar

1 teaspoon sriracha (optional; see notes)

1 teaspoon sucanat or other sweetener

1. Put everything into the bowl of a food processor fitted with the s-shaped metal blade. Process until smooth.

2. Taste and adjust seasonings if necessary.

notes

Sriracha is a Vietnamese condiment made from garlic and chiles. It's great to keep around if you like spicy food.

See the note on the previous page about alternatives to a food processor.

(cont.)

variations

- You can leave out the tofu for a thinner, sharper sauce; that also makes it into a good tofu *topping*.

lisa p.'s crack spice rub

My friend Lisa P. gave me this recipe. I don't know where she got it, but it really is as addictive as the name suggests. I think it's the sugar. She makes it as Cauliflower Crack. I like to mix it up a little more, with combinations of different veggies, and bring it to potlucks, so that's the main recipe I'm giving you. Think about putting it on anything, though.

🕐 Takes 20 to 25 minutes and serves eight to 10 as a side dish.

2 teaspoons paprika

2 teaspoons cumin

1 teaspoon cinnamon

1 dash cayenne (to taste)

1 teaspoon sucanat or other granulated sweetener

½ teaspoon sea salt (see the note about salt textures and
     measurements in the pantry section)

2 tablespoons olive oil (or more if necessary)

2 pounds sweet-friendly vegetables like cauliflower, sweet
     potatoes, carrots, parsnips, beets, and/or regular
     potatoes (NOT bitter-ish green veggies, like broccoli or
     brussels sprouts), prepped for roasting (see page 76)

1. Preheat oven to 450°F.

2. Put the chopped veggies in a big plastic container or lidded bowl with the oil and all the spices and sugar. Shake it all up until everything's evenly coated with spices and oil. Roast for 20 minutes, stirring halfway through (see Roasted Vegetables, page 76,

for more information on all this; the temperature is a little lower here because the intense browning that you want on plain veggies can make spices bitter and burnt-tasting).

variations

• Try the spice rub on tempeh: Omit the sweetener, replace the salt with a tablespoon of soy sauce, and cut the oil to a scant tablespoon. Cut a package of tempeh into bite-size pieces. Combine everything and shake to coat as described in step 2, above. Sauté over medium high heat in a skillet or griddle pan until crispy and browned on the outside and heated through. The oil should provide enough for the frying, but you can coat the pan if you think you need it. (See Debbie's Tempeh, page 69, for more info.)

• Try switching up the spice combo: try cumin, coriander, ground chiles, curry powder, on both vegetables and tempeh, with and without sugar as you see fit.

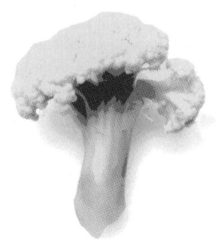

citrus vinaigrette for any salad

As with so many of my favorite recipes, I learned the basic method for this endlessly flexible dressing from Deborah Madison's *Vegetarian Cooking for Everyone*. You can put anything in it, you can put it on anything. I've got some suggestions below, but don't even think about letting them limit you. Oh, and, technically it's not a vinaigrette, because it's not actually made with vinegar. Whatever.

⏱ Takes less than 10 minutes to make the dressing. Serves a totally flexible number of people depending on your salad, how juicy your citrus is, and how tart you like your vinaigrette. Salads themselves tend not to keep all that well, but the dressing itself will keep for more than a week, in case you don't use it all.

2 lemons or limes

1 clove minced garlic, 1 tablespoon minced shallot, ½ tablespoon minced onion, 1½ tablespoons finely chopped chives, or 1 finely chopped scallion (basically, any member of the allium family, minced or chopped, in a small quantity depending on its strength)

¼ cup olive oil (this can't be anything but approximate; however much you need depends too much on your taste and the amount of juice that came out of the citrus)

½ teaspoon dijon mustard (see note)

1 small handful parsley, finely chopped (optional; you could also use any fresh or dried herb you have on hand that you think would go with your salad items)

salt and pepper to taste

1. Zest one of your citruses into a jelly jar or other small container with a lid that closes securely (this makes it much easier because you can just shake to mix, but if all you've got's a bowl, use that). Juice both citruses into the jar.

2. Mince or chop whatever allium you're using (if it's garlic, mash it into a paste with the side of your knife after chopping). Add it to juice and zest.

3. Add the mustard if you're using it, along with salt and pepper and any herbs (if you're using fresh herbs and you're not going to dress the salad soon, wait until right before to add them). Shake it all up. Taste and adjust the amount of oil and seasoning. Cold food generally needs a little more salt than hot food, and don't forget that your dressing is going to be spread out over a lot of stuff.

note

The mustard acts as an emulsifier, keeping the oil and the water (in the form of juice) more integrated. So although you can leave it out, a better option if you won't want a mustard flavor is to use dry mustard instead of dijon.

variations

■ Like I said, this is endlessly flexible. Some suggestions: Cooled roasted beets (see the roasting instructions, page 76) on their own or with baby spinach or other dark greens; mint (and/or feta if you go for that kind of thing) would also be a nice addition to that combo. Corn, tomatoes, and garbanzo beans are lovely together. Blanched snap peas, green beans, or asparagus are great on their own or in combination with other things. If your usual food-shopping haunts have them, try leafy sprouts like buckwheat, pea, or sunflower, along with usual salad suspects such as tomatoes, cucumbers, celery, carrots, and bell peppers.

As you can tell, I'm not crazy about regular lettuce-based salads, but of course you can dress lettuce with this, and add lettuce to anything you think it would be good in.

Also, if you don't have any tart citrus around, you can also make this using any kind of vinegar your little heart desires (or keeps in its cabinet).

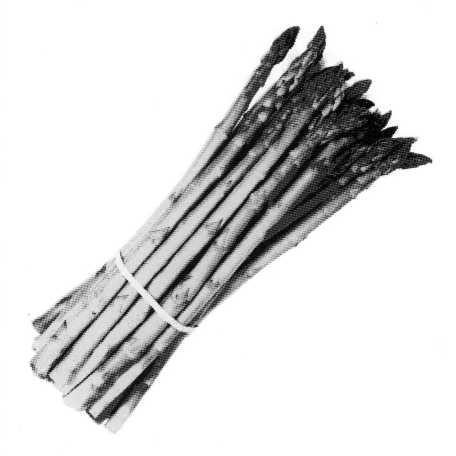

citrus vinaigrette for any salad

corn and tomato salad

This is a great contribution to a summer potluck or picnic. With some good crusty whole-grain bread, it also makes a good light meal when you're too hot to deal with much of anything else.

🕐 Takes about 20 minutes. Serves four and doubles well.

3 ears corn

1 large tomato or two medium, three small, or one basket of cherry tomatoes

1 small handful fresh basil, roughly chopped or torn

1 lemon (you'll want the zest and the juice)

2 tablespoons olive oil (or more/less to taste)

salt and pepper to taste

1. Husk the corn and steam it for five or so minutes in an inch or two of boiling salted water, turning once or twice. (This is quicker and easier than a full boil and just as effective.)

2. Cool the corn in a bowl of ice water or in the freezer until it's cool enough to handle (read about carryover cooking in "Tips and Techniques," page 39). Cut the kernels off the cobs and cool further if necessary.

3. Cut the tomatoes into bite-size pieces and put them in a bowl with the corn and the basil. (If you're using cherry tomatoes, cut the larger ones in half and keep the smaller ones whole.)

4. Zest half the lemon into the bowl (you really don't need all the zest, that would be too much). Juice the lemon into the bowl (don't work too hard to get everything out of it; you want to have

some left in case you want to add it to adjust the flavors after the oil is added).

5. Pour the olive oil over everything. Toss to coat. Taste and adjust the lemon/oil balance, adding whichever is necessary. Add salt and pepper to taste.

variations

• Obviously, quantities are quite flexible. This could be turned into a main-course pasta salad with the addition of some leftover or cooked and cooled penne or shells (it might take two lemons and four tablespoons of oil for the dressing, depending on quantities).

• You could also add other things (cubes of fresh mozzarella come to mind for the non-vegans among us), but I really like to keep it simple. Check out Citrus Vinaigrette for Any Salad, page 91, for other ideas for lemon vinaigrette.

• It could also become a wholly different animal as a corn and cucumber salad, with limes and mint replacing the lemons and basil.

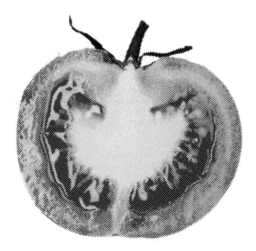

lime-cumin summer salad

This is my absolute favorite thing to bring to a potluck or serve at a party in the summertime. It all started when I first made Deborah Madison's lime-cumin vinaigrette from *Vegetarian Cooking for Everyone* and it inspired all sorts of ideas about what it would taste perfect on. The salad is different every time I make it, because there are so many vegetable/grain/bean combos that work so beautifully. The dressing is a streamlined and simplified version of the original inspiration.

⏱ Takes about 35 minutes. Serves six as a side, though it's endlessly expandable (see note) and can easily become a main course (see variations). It keeps well, flavorwise, but old salad veggies can get...old.

for the dressing:

2 limes (you'll want the zest from one and the juice from both)

1 small clove garlic (or half a large one)

1 pinch sea salt, plus more to taste

2 scallions, both white and green parts, sliced into very thin rings or finely chopped

½ a jalapeño pepper, seeds and ribs removed, minced

1½ teaspoons ground cumin

¾ teaspoon coriander

¼ teaspoon dry mustard (you can use wet mustard if it's the only thing you have, though it will add a bit of vinegar flavor, or leave it out)

¼ cup olive oil (as with all dressings, I can only estimate
   here due to differences in taste and differences between
   limes; you'll just need to keep adding more and tasting
   until it has your preferred balance of oil with lime juice)
1 small handful cilantro, finely chopped

for the salad:

4 ears corn
1 large cucumber, peeled if the skin is bitter, and sliced into
   quarter-rounds
1 small bunch radishes (about five or six)
2 large handfuls of cherry tomatoes (cut the big ones in half
   and leave the small ones whole); if you don't have or
   don't want to use cherry tomatoes, use full-size ones cut
   into bite-size pieces
1 large handful green beans, stems removed and cut into
   1- to 2-inch pieces
1 cup cooked barley

1. If you want to use barley and you don't have any left over from
something else, get that going first. (See "Tips and Techniques,"
page 39, for grain-cooking instructions, including cooling grains
for salad and the timing of dressing them.)

2. Next, prepare the veggies that need to be cooked. Bring a
few inches of water to a boil in a sauté pan or stockpot (anything,
really, as long as it has a tight-fitting lid); husk the corn and stick
the ears in there (you can break them if they don't fit). Cook for
about five minutes, turning the ears so that no one part ends up

lime-cumin summer salad

submerged in water the whole time. Remove from pan and stick in a bowl of ice water (read about carryover cooking in "Tips and Techniques," page 39). Put your green beans in a steamer basket and put it in the pan you used for the corn (see what a neat trick that is, not having to boil new water?); cover tightly. (If you don't have a steamer basket, you can put them right in the water; just know that they'll cook much faster.) Cook until bright green and tender (about five to seven minutes, but it really depends on quantity and whether the basket is tightly packed, so check often). Cool them in a bowl of ice water, too (you did go read about carryover cooking, right?).

3. Zest one of the limes into a jelly jar or other small container with a lid that closes securely (this makes it much easier because you can just shake to mix, but if all you've got's a bowl, use that). Juice both limes into your jar.

4. Mince the garlic; then, sprinkle some salt on top and smush it into a paste with the side of your knife. Add it to the lime juice and zest.

5. Add everything else except the cilantro, close your tight-fitting lid, and shake vigorously. Taste; add more oil and salt if necessary, little by little. Do that until it tastes right, keeping in mind that the flavors and salt will be spread over the whole salad, so it should be on the salty side.

6. If you're going to dress the salad right away, add the cilantro now; if not, wait until about 15 minutes before you're going to pour the dressing on. Set aside and the flavors will meld. (You can make the dressing several days in advance if you want.)

7. Assemble the salad: Cut the corn off the cob and put it in a big bowl with all the other veggies and the cooled barley. Add the

dressing no more than an hour before you plan to eat (well, okay, you can add it whenever you want and it will still taste good, but adding it too far in advance can lead to a bit of veggie wilting; if you want to do things in advance, you can make the dressing and assemble the salad the day before and store them separately). Because the quantities in the recipe are pretty general, it's a good idea to add the dressing in parts so you don't drown the salad. Just toss and taste along the way.

note

The number of servings you'll get depends, obviously, on the variations and how much of what you put in. It's easy to stretch this for a crowd (if you're trying to feed 10 or more, add another lime and extra oil, and use a slightly heavier hand with the spices (heaping teaspoons rather than level ones).

variations

• In the dressing, everything but the limes, spices, and either garlic or scallions (though you could use shallots, red onion, or chives) is optional. If you leave things out, your flavors will be less complex but still good. Cilantro could also be replaced with parsley for a milder vibe.

• In the salad itself, literally every ingredient is replaceable. The ones I listed here make up my favorite combination of easy-to-find veggies, but you can use practically anything: any combination of what's listed along with or substituted with bell peppers of all colors, steamed or raw snap peas or snow peas, raw shelled English peas, carrots, jicama, celery–if it sounds good to you, chances are it will be. You can use rice, couscous, or quinoa instead of barley, or have no grain at all. If you're using couscous or quinoa, under-cook it just a tad/go light on the water to minimize the chance of mushiness. To make it a main course or just give it some extra heartiness, throw in a can of drained and rinsed black beans.

greens pie with herbs and lemon

This is one of the more complicated things in this book, and I even debated leaving it out because it doesn't really fit the simple/no planning vibe I'm trying to cultivate. But I love it, and it's a really great thing to serve company or bring to a potluck. It's good hot and at room temperature, and you can make it in advance up to the baking step.

🕐 Takes just over an hour, but for half of that it's in the oven, so you don't really have to do anything during that time. Serves six to eight. Extra good with roasted potatoes on the side.

1 bunch spinach or ½ pound baby spinach leaves

2 bunches kale (dino, a.k.a. lacinto, preferred), destemmed and chopped

1 bunch scallions, both white and green parts, sliced into thin rounds

2 small handfuls parsley, chopped

1 small handful cilantro, chopped

1½ tablespoons olive oil, plus a little more to grease the pan

1½ teaspoons sea salt (split between greens and tofu mixture; also, see the note about salt textures and measurements in the pantry section)

1 lemon (you'll want both the zest and the juice)

1 12-ounce package firm tofu (this is a pretty standard package size; I do suggest staying as close to that as possible or your pie might feel light on greens)

(cont.)

½ cup soy yogurt

¼ cup nutritional yeast

pepper to taste

1. Preheat the oven to 375°F.

2. Wilt the spinach in a skillet or sauté pan over low to medium heat: Just toss it in there, no oil or water needed; cover it and the moisture in the spinach will be all you need. Stir it or turn with tongs to distribute the heat and keep it from burning. When all the leaves are wilted, put the spinach in a colander to cool. When it's no longer too hot to handle, squeeze as much water out of it as you can.

3. In the meantime, heat the oil over medium heat (it's easiest to use the same pan you used for the spinach; no need to wash it). Add the scallions, kale, parsley, cilantro, and one teaspoon of the salt. Cook until the kale is wilted and the scallions are tender (about 10 to 15 minutes).

4. Put the kale mixture into a bowl with the squeezed spinach. Zest the lemon into the bowl; then cut the lemon in half and squeeze its juice in, too. Set aside.

5. Put the tofu, soy yogurt, nutritional yeast, and ½ teaspoon salt into the bowl of a food processor fitted with the s-shaped metal blade and whir until smooth.

6. Stir the tofu mixture into the greens with some fresh-ground pepper. Taste it and add more salt and/or whatever else you think it needs.

7. Oil a baking pan (9-inch round or square works best) and press the mixture into it. Bake for 40 minutes or so–the top should

be good and golden brown, and you'll be able to see that the tofu has gotten kinda puffed up.

note

If you don't have a food processor, you can mix your soy and stuff up with a stick blender, a hand mixer, or a wooden spoon, though the texture will not be as smooth (especially with the spoon option).

variations

- You can use any combination of greens (spinach, all kale varieties, chard, collards, beet greens, turnip greens)—you'll need about two pounds total. Spinach is the only one you need to squeeze the water out of; everything else should be treated like the kale. Also, if you use all spinach, you'll need more like three pounds, since it cooks down so much due to the water content.

- You can also swap out the cilantro for other herbs—try different herb/greens combinations that sound good to you.

- You can substitute leeks, green garlic (which is garlic harvested early, before it splits into so many cloves; it also has usable stems like a scallion), spring onions, shallots, or regular onions for the scallions.

- You can fancy it up by baking it in a pie crust or wrapped in phyllo (see the method outlined in "Tips and Techniques," page 39).

oatmeal-fruit cookies

One of the many times I made these for a party at my house, a guest stopped in the middle of her sentence to remark on the obscene amount of butter that must be in them. When I told her that they had no butter or eggs at all, she didn't believe me until I actually gave her the recipe. Her boyfriend said he wanted to start a cookie business using it, but, unfortunately, he was all talk.

Some of the ingredient distinctions may seem fussy, and you're right, they kinda are. As listed, they give the best flavor and texture even if it is annoying to go out and buy two kinds of oats and two kinds of flour. You don't absolutely have to, though; read through the variations to see what your options for simplifying things are. Also possibly fussy-seeming is the fact that some of the ingredient quantities are given in weight in addition to volume. There's a good reason for this, though, and you'll have much more consistency and better results if you use the weight measurements—measuring cups are notoriously inaccurate for dry ingredients; a cup of flour can vary by more than half an ounce, depending on how you get the flour into the cup. But if you don't have a scale, go with the volumes and know that your results may vary (read up on this at www.baking911.com/howto/measure.htm if you so desire). The recipe is adapted from an extremely non-vegan one I learned when I took a five-day intensive baking class at the Culinary Institute of America.

⏱ Takes about 20 minutes to make the dough and 15 minutes to bake each sheet of cookies (see notes). This recipe makes about six dozen cookies, though, so the whole project usually takes almost two hours.

⅓ cup walnut oil

⅓ cup canola oil (see the footnote about canola on page 32)

17¼ ounces (3 cups) sucanat or evaporated cane juice

6 tablespoons soft silken tofu

3 tablespoons applesauce (should be unsweetened and free of added flavorings)

1 tablespoon prune puree (see notes)

½ tablespoon vanilla extract

4½ ounces (1 cup) all-purpose whole wheat flour

4¼ ounces (1 scant cup) whole wheat pastry flour

½ teaspoon sea salt (see the note about salt texture and measurements in the pantry section)

½ teaspoon baking soda

½ tablespoon cinnamon

6 ounces (1¾ cups) rolled oats (neither quick-cooking nor instant)

5¼ ounces (1½ cups) quick-cooking rolled oats (not instant)

4 ounces (¾ cup) chopped dried apricots (unsulphured and unsweetened)

4 ounces (¾ cup) chopped dried cherries (unsulphured and unsweetened)

4 ounces (¾ cup) dried cranberries (they are generally already chopped or just small enough not to need chopping; unsweetened and unsulphured if possible, though that can be very hard to find)

1. Preheat oven to 350°F.

2. With a hand mixer (or a wooden spoon), beat the oil and

sucanat in a large bowl at high speed until the sugar is dissolved and you've gotten some air in there.

3. Combine the tofu, applesauce, prune puree, and vanilla in a small bowl and mix well. You don't need to worry about getting them totally combined because you're about to beat the whole thing into the oil/sugar mixture, but you do want to get them pretty well mushed together.

4. Beat the tofu mixture into the oil and sugar at high speed for a couple minutes. Any remaining bits of tofu should be pretty damn tiny.

5. Put the mixer away; it's all spoons from here on out. Mix the flour, salt, baking soda, and cinnamon together in a medium bowl. Stir the results into the oil/sugar mixture, using as few strokes as possible, until reasonably well combined.

6. Add the oats and stir (again with as few strokes as possible) until no streaks of flour or oats are left. Add the dried fruit and stir to distribute.

7. Scoop by tablespoons onto a baking sheet lined with parchment paper and bake for 15 minutes (or until lightly browned on the bottom). Let the cookies cool on the sheet for a few minutes before removing to a cooling rack. (If you don't have parchment paper, grease your sheet with a little oil and start checking for doneness a few minutes early.)

notes

I think it's best to do one sheet at a time, but you can try it with two if you swap the sheet positions halfway through and are prepared improvise on the baking time—they will likely take at least two minutes longer, maybe more.

oatmeal-fruit cookies

Make prune puree in a food processor fitted with an s-shaped metal blade by whirring together equal parts prunes and water. It keeps for a long time in the fridge. It's really useful in this recipe, but you can leave it out and add a tad more applesauce instead.

variations

• If dealing with two kinds of oil, two kinds of flour, and two kinds of oats is too much hoo-ha for you (and to be honest it's often too much for me), to make it simpler and easier, any of the following substitutions can be made: all regular rolled oats rather than part quick oats; all pastry flour instead of part all-purpose flour (or vice versa); white flour for whole wheat flour, brown or white sugar for the sucanat (though please note that, because of the vast difference in sugar textures, you really have to measure the sugar by weight if you're making a substitution). For the oil, you can use all canola, all walnut, or any combination of neutral-tasting vegetable oil and nut oil; I like the walnut/canola combo the best because it has a buttery flavor. You'll get slightly different textures depending on what you use, and the baking times will vary as well, so keep a close eye on your cookies' progress.

• You can vary the flavor with different dried fruits. You can use any fruits in any combinations, as long as they add up to 12 ounces (or approximately 2¼ cups chopped): apricots, cherries, nectarines, peaches, pears, apples, blueberries, strawberries, raisins, currants. The combination in the main recipe is my favorite, though, and (surprise!) I have some other opinions: It's best to have at least four ounces of cranberries for tartness no matter what; dried strawberries are too sweet and make things taste kinda jammy; dried apples are spongy; dried blueberries are expensive and usually don't taste like much (plus they usually have added sweetener); raisins and currants tend to overwhelm the other fruits and give kind of a boring (or, if you like it, classic) flavor. But, hey, they're you're cookies when you make them, so go to town.

- You can also experiment with adding nuts, or swapping the cinnamon for other spices, such as nutmeg (much stronger than cinnamon, so a little goes a long way), cardamom, allspice, or ground ginger (try using a small amount of candied ginger for some of the fruit).

spicy brownies

I spent several years on a quest for the perfect brownie. I tasted a lot of chocolate, tested a lot of recipes, fed a lot of friends substandard brownies, and learned a ton from the trial and error. And, in my not-so-humble opinion, I succeeded in my quest. And then I changed it all again for the veganish whole-foods thing. This is the result. See Oatmeal-Fruit Cookies, page 104, for a discussion of weight versus volume in cooking measurements.

⏱ Takes about an hour and 10 minutes (50 of which are baking). Makes between nine and 16 brownies depending on how big you cut 'em.

4 ounces bittersweet chocolate with as close to 72 percent cocoa as you can find (see notes)

4 tablespoons canola oil (see the footnote about canola on page 32)

½ cup brown rice syrup

¾ cup sucanat or evaporated cane juice

2 tablespoons applesauce

2 tablespoons soft silken tofu

½ tablespoon prune puree (optional)

2 teaspoons vanilla extract

4½ ounces (1 cup) whole wheat flour

1 ounce (¼ cup) cocoa powder

¼ teaspoon sea salt (see the note about salt textures and measurements in the pantry section)

1 teaspoon cinnamon

a scant ⅛ teaspoon cayenne pepper

1. Preheat the oven to 350°F.

2. Melt the bittersweet chocolate with the canola oil in a bowl set on top of a pan of simmering water over low heat (see notes). If the bowl used for melting isn't big enough to accommodate all the ingredients, remove to a large bowl when melted and set aside to cool slightly.

3. In a small bowl, thoroughly mix the applesauce, tofu, and prune puree; set aside.

4. Add the rice syrup, sucanat, and vanilla to the chocolate mixture. Mix well.

5. Mix the tofu/applesauce into the chocolate/sugar.

6. Mix the flour, cocoa powder, salt, cinnamon, and cayenne together in a medium bowl. Add them to the rest of the batter and stir to just combine.

7. Pour it all into a parchment-lined or oiled 9-inch square baking pan.

8. Bake for 50 minutes or until a toothpick inserted into the center comes out with only crumbs (no wet batter) sticking to it. Cool in the pan, preferably on a rack, for 10 to 15 minutes. Turn it out of the pan to cool completely (also preferably on a rack) before cutting into squares.

notes

The quality of your chocolate matters. If you start with so-so chocolate, your brownies will never be any better than so-so. I use Schokinag bittersweet bars, which have 72 percent cocoa solids, and Schokinag cocoa powder. They can be hard to find, though, so if you're not up for a hunt and/or ordering chocolate off the internet, then just use something *good* with a cocoa solid percentage as close to 72 as possible (that number affects how much fat and sugar is in the chocolate as well, and the recipe is formulated to have a certain amount of both of those items in total).

When melting the chocolate, the key is not to put it over direct heat. Chocolate needs gradual, gentle heat. This is what double-boilers are made for, so in the unlikely event you have one, use it. But since no one has double-boilers anymore (and why should they?), just use a bowl resting over (better) or sitting in (still okay) a pan of simmering water.

variations

- Orange brownies: Omit the cinnamon and cayenne. Replace the vanilla with orange flower water or orange liqueur (optional). Add the zest of an orange along with the rice syrup and sucanat.

- Black forest brownies: Omit the cinnamon and cayenne. Replace the vanilla with kirsch (cherry brandy). Stir in ½ cup dried cherries (chopped if they're big) after the flour.

- Experiment with different flavors of extracts and different dried fruits, nuts, or chocolate chips. Just omit the cinnamon and cayenne, use any liquid flavorings to replace the vanilla, and add solids at the very end, after the flour.

- You can also make these plain by just omitting the cinnamon and cayenne. Boring but still delicious.

spicy brownies

nonrecipe recipes
(a.k.a., ideas for snacks and meals that are too easy to be called recipes)

THE KEY TO CONSISTENT HEALTHY EATING IS TO KEEP THINGS on hand that you can snack on or prepare easily. Not every meal has to be a full-blown home-cooked one to be good and satisfying, and some packaged foods, most notably salad dressings, sauces, and spreads can be incredibly useful in making it easier to eat fresh whole foods when you're pressed for time (just read the labels to find the ones without food additives, corn syrup, and artificial colors and flavors).

breakfast

My favorite breakfast is **steel-cut oats** made in my rice cooker: I just put one part oats, four and a half parts water, and a generous pinch of salt into the cooker on the porridge setting right when I wake up, and by the time I'm finished with my morning routine, it's ready. (If I'm gonna be in a hurry in the morning, I'll increase the water a bit and do it the night before.) You can top it with anything that sounds good to you: fruit, nuts, cinnamon, ground cardamom, maple syrup, almond milk, whatever. (If you're going to use cinnamon or any other spice, though, you probably want to put it in the rice cooker instead of sprinkling it on top afterwards.)

I like mine with olive oil, mixed dried fruit, walnuts, and roasted cocoa nibs, but if I'm out of any of those things it's still great with less. You can also **try other grains** (I like quinoa in the morning) or mixed-grain cereals in your local bulk section.

The **toast + spread** routine below can also work well first thing in the morning.

snacks

The easiest snack of all is something you can just pull out of the fridge or cupboard and eat: **fresh fruit, or vegetables that can be eaten raw** (carrots, celery, cucumbers, bell peppers). **Nuts and dried fruit** are also great easy snacks, plus they generally stay good for as long as it takes to eat them (if you're slow with nuts, put 'em in the fridge to stave off rancidity).

For a larger snack that actually qualifies as a light lunch, I always have on hand some whole-grain bread that lasts a while in the fridge (my current favorite is Vital Vittles Russian sourdough). In summer, I get tomatoes and quark (a soft yogurt-based cheese) from the farmers market to put on top; in winter it's usually hummus and carrots, since there are no tomatoes. This routine is endlessly adaptable: **toast + spread** (hummus, peanut or other nut butter, pesto, soft cheese, whatever you like) **+ vegetable or fruit** that goes with your spread (cucumbers, bell peppers, spinach, apples)–just spread, slice, stack, and eat.

lunch and dinner

You can make a **main-course salad** in about 10 minutes (20 if you need to steam or blanch things) with whatever veggies you have on hand, a can of beans (I like garbanzos best for salads) or some sprouted beans if you can get 'em (both of the farmers markets I go to regularly have a vendor that sells sprouted lentils, sprouted bean mix, and the like), and a shot of dressing from a bottle. Those packages of smoked spiced tofu can supplement or replace the beans, and if you have a little more time you can make a quick dressing (like the citrus vinaigrette on page 91, or just by shaking together some oil, some vinegar, and whatever other flavors you might want [and maybe a bit of mustard to help with the emulsifying]). As long as the flavors of what you're using seem appealing to you, you're set.

It's also incredibly easy to put together a meal with **pasta or rice** (especially if you have a rice cooker that you can load up in the morning for fresh hot rice upon your return home). Either of these can be **topped with some simple flavoring items**: olive oil and parmesan cheese or nutritional yeast; sautéed garlic, if you're feeling like using a skillet; jarred tomato sauce; or a drizzle each of sesame oil, soy sauce, and hot chili oil (if you like spicy), with a dash of nutritional yeast; or, as mentioned above, some kind of relatively unprocessed bottled sauce, dressing, or marinade that appeals to you (I like peanut sauce even when I'm too busy to make my own). To **add a little vegetable** (always a good idea, in my opinion), you can chop a tomato and toss it on there (no need to cook it at all; I would only do this with the oil and/or garlic or tomato sauce, but not with the sesame oil flavorings), or chop some spinach and either add it to your bowl of hot starch (the heat from the already-hot food will wilt it) or, if you're using pasta, put it in the colander and drain the pasta over it, which will cook it more thoroughly than wilting it in the bowl. You can also toss broccoli florets, green beans, or some other needs-a-bit-of-time-to-cook veggie in with the pasta or on top of still-cooking rice at the last minute. (Of course, if you have a rice cooker and so your rice is just keeping warm already, you'll have to sauté, steam, or blanch your veggies separately; see "Tips and Techniques," page 39. If you're using a rice cooker and your rice is still going, you can put veggies in on top, but there are a couple caveats with that. One is that rice cooker cooking times are often different from stovetop cooking times, and not all rice cookers will tell you how much time is left, so it can be hard to know when to put the veggies in. The other is that many rice cookers use some sort of sensor technology involving moisture or weight to tell when the grain is done. So putting veggies in there might throw things off.)

You can also press the water out of some **tofu** (see "Tips and Techniques" again), fry up the slabs in a little oil in a skillet or griddle pan, and pour some of those bottled sauces mentioned above on top. Pair it with some vegetables cooked in the same griddle pan (see Ginger-Garlic-Sesame Tofu with Spinach, page 64), or separately (see "Tips and Techniques" yet again).

See how easy it is to make a quick, wholesome, tasty meal?

further resources

reading

A highly incomplete, quirky-as-I-am list of suggested in-depth reading on the issues I touch on superficially.

- *Animal, Vegetable, Miracle: A Year of Food Life*, by Barbara Kingsolver, Camille Kingsolver, and Steven L. Hopp (Harper Perennial). Acclaimed novelist Barbara Kingsolver and her family spent a year growing most of their own food and getting the rest from other local farmers, and then they wrote this book about it. Barbara provides the narrative (and after reading it, you definitely feel part of her life enough to call her by her first name); her daughter Camille contributes recipes; and her husband Steven contributes informative (though brief and thus not in-depth) sidebars on things like pesticide usage and heirloom seeds. What powerfully distinguishes *Animal, Vegetable, Miracle* from other accounts of local eating is the Kingsolver-Hopp clan's level of commitment—they'd been planning a cross-country move to a house where they could have a small-scale farm for years, long before local eating became a popular memoir topic. This book is about their lives, not an experiment.

- *Diet for a Dead Planet: How the Food Industry Is Killing Us*, by Christopher Cook (New Press). Cook's sharp exposé of how corporate capitalism and industrial agriculture wreak havoc on workers, the environment, and our health is depressing and galvanizing at the same time. You just have to read it. Seriously.

- The Ethicurean (www.ethicurean.com). With the tagline "Chew the right thing," this multiauthor blog features news and commentary on food policy in the U.S. and globally, food safety, sustainability, food-related labor issues, and more. It's the best way I've found to keep up with the latest goings on in the world from an ethical-food perspective, though the volume can feel overwhelming at times.

- *Food Fight: The Citizen's Guide to a Food and Farm Bill*, by Daniel Imhoff (University of California Press). Published in 2007, before the latest version of the farm bill was finalized, *Food Fight* is nonetheless a relevant and useful primer on what you need to know and why you should care about the ins and outs of policies that can make your eyes glaze over.

- *Food Politics: How the Food Industry Influences Nutrition and Health*, by Marion Nestle (University of California Press). Nestle, a professor of nutrition and public health, is a tireless advocate for real food and sensible eating. Her 2002 exposé is *the* source for how agribusiness and food manufacturers hold sway over U.S. food and nutrition policies. You'll be shocked and appalled—and, hopefully, moved to make some change.

- *In Defense of Food: An Eater's Manifesto*, by Michael Pollan (Penguin). Michael Pollan is my hero. This slim volume enumerating everything that's wrong with what passes for food in U.S.

supermarkets, and suggesting some simple rules for better eating, is a tad on the dry side but still excellent.

• *The Omnivore's Dilemma: A Natural History of Four Meals*, by Michael Pollan (Penguin). One of the most accessible and enjoyable books around on where your food comes from and why it matters. Structured (as the subtitle hints) around the ingredients in a fast-food meal, a Whole Foods meal, a meal where everything comes from one spectacularly sustainable farm in Virginia, and one meal in which Pollan himself hunts and forages as much of dinner as possible, *The Omnivore's Dilemma* is an entertaining and in-depth introduction to major topics in food politics.

• *The Revolution Will Not Be Microwaved: Inside America's Underground Food Movements*, by Sandor Ellix Katz (Chelsea Green). Longtime foodie zinester Katz, author of the also-awesome *Wild Fermentation* (see the canning and preserving section below), visits raw milk producers, foragers, and seed savers and explores the connections among food, health, land stewardship, labor struggles, and more. This engaging and politically astute synthesis will make you want to go out and find all the folks in your area who are working to strengthen and expand local food systems and traditional foodways.

• *Stuffed and Starved: The Hidden Battle for the World's Food System*, by Raj Patel (Melville House). Critically examining globalized food markets, government and institutional food policy, corporate seed company shenanigans, and much, much more, *Stuffed and Starved* lays out some absolutely essential pieces of the food system puzzle. Want to know how the International Monetary Fund contributes to famine? Want to understand farmer suicides in Korea and India? It helps to already have some knowledge of these issues when you start reading, because Patel is so deep in his material that he doesn't always stop to spell everything out, but that's a minor flaw in a work that simply must be read. Without it, you can't have a full understanding of the magnitude and scope of the systemic problems we all face.

• *The Way We Eat: Why Our Food Choices Matter*, by Peter Singer and Jim Mason (Rodale). Through profiles of three families with different eating styles, Singer, a philosophy professor and ethicist famous for the 1975 instant classic *Animal Liberation*, and his writing partner research and engage questions like "Is local always more environmental?," "What does free range mean?," and "Is humane meat possible?" More philosophically rigorous (and more of a polemic) than *The Omnivore's Dilemma*, it's an only slightly less fascinating read.

cooking

These are cookbooks I draw inspiration from, think have good nutritional or philosophical information, or just find useful. Also highly subjective, extremely incomplete, and not all vegan or vegetarian.

• *Another Dinner Is Possible*, by the Anarchist Teapot Mobile Kitchen (kinda hard to figure out who the publisher actually is, but I got my copy from Microcosm Publishing, www.microcosmpub lishing.com). Written by a lefty British catering collective, this is admittedly not the most useful book for a U.S. resident, what with the unfamiliar terminology and the metric measurements. But it's got a mix of straightforward and downright weird recipes that make good fodder for mulling over the question of what you feel like making for dinner. (And if you want to read some very grassroots essays on peak oil, eating disorders, and eating vegan while pregnant, you're in luck.)

- Epicurious.com's advanced search function (http://www. epicurious.com/recipesmenus/advancedsearch). This is so useful I don't even care that it's brought to us by corporate glossy magazine behemoth Condé Nast. You can search by keyword, preparation method, course, occasion, and more—and, at the same time, check boxes for vegetarian, vegan, quick, kosher, kid-friendly, nut-free: pretty much anything you can think of. So when you have, say, rutabagas in your CSA box and you don't know what to do with them, you know where to go. Reader ratings and comments offer useful tips for variations and improvements.

- *Get It Ripe*, by Jae Steele (Arsenal Pulp Press). Steele is a nutritionist, and her approach is a little bit fussy for my taste, with a risk of making you feel like a failure if you don't incorporate into your daily routine the proper amounts of a long list of micronutrients. She also strongly cautions you not to change a thing in your preparation of her recipes, which, if you've read anything in this book, is an instruction that you already know I don't think is worth following. That said, she's got good information and inventive, tasty recipes, so it's well worth getting past the attitude.

- *Grub: Ideas for an Urban Organic Kitchen*, by Anna Lappé and Bryant Terry (Jeremy P. Tarcher/Penguin). Even more than the full menu-planned recipes, I appreciate this book for its accessible yet comprehensive overview of all the political and health reasons to eat real food, plus the concrete "Seven Steps to a Grub Kitchen" chapter, including budget tips.

- *The Healthy Hedonist*, by Myra Kornfeld (Simon & Schuster). Most cookbooks that reference health in their titles are all about fat reduction and whatnot. Kornfeld is all about whole foods, and she is awesome. Her additive-free onion dip recipes (she has three versions, one of which is vegan) have already made many of my friends deliriously happy. And her sweet potato and red pepper spread recipe alone is worth the price of the book. I'd be shocked if you didn't find a bunch of dishes you'll be eager to try just by paging through.

- *The Roasted Vegetable*, by Andrea Chesman (Harvard Common Press). The name pretty much says it all: tons of recipes using roasted vegetables. This can mean a lot of steps (when I roast vegetables, I tend to just want to eat them, not keep cooking so I can add them to something else), but if you're up for a bit of a project, it's going to be totally worth it.

- *Super Natural Cooking*, by Heidi Swanson (Celestial Arts). This might be the most beautiful cookbook I have ever seen. It's certainly the most beautiful one I own. Subtitled "Five Ways to Incorporate Whole & Natural Ingredients into Your Cooking," it's as much about strategies and ingredients as it is about the recipes themselves, so even if you never make risotto-style barley with winter citrus and arugula (though oh my gawd, how can you not want to?), *Super Natural Cooking* will serve you very, very well.

- *Sustainable Eating*'s recipe archive (www.semagazine.com/recipearchive.php). This online magazine ceased publication in 2007, but the recipe archive remains a small but valuable source of simple, seasonal cooking ideas.

- *Vegan on a Shoestring*, by the People's Potato Project Collective (self-published by the collective, peoplespotato.blogspot.com; available through Microcosm, www.microcosmpublishing.com). The People's Potato is a soup kitchen serving students and activists at Concordia University in Montreal, Canada. They give a great overview of basic cooking techniques and simple, appealing recipes. And if you ever need to make a tasty, nutritious meal for a small army of protesters, they have a whole section on cooking for a crowd. Plus: cute illustrations.

- *Vegan with a Vengeance*, by Isa Chandra Moskowitz, and *Veganomicon*, by Isa Chandra Moskowitz and Terry Hope Romero (Marlowe and Company). These are vegan bibles, because Isa Moskowitz and Terry Romero, her co-conspirator on the public access TV show *Post Punk Kitchen*, are pretty genius with the vegan versions of familiar foods. They're not really on the whole-foods tip, so I tend not to cook from their books all that much (plus they have a penchant for labor-intensive individual preparations, like spring rolls and empanadas, that try my patience, but that's just me)—but I still find them indispensable for menu ideas, for veganizing techniques, and just to read, because they're totally fun.

- *Vegetarian Cooking for Everyone*, by Deborah Madison (Broadway Books). This is an indispensable addition to your cookbook library, no matter what your eating style. It has 1,200 recipes. I haven't cooked every last one, but everything I have cooked has been delicious. If I had to, I could cook only from this book for the rest of my life; if I were picking one cookbook to take with me to the desert island, yup, this is the one. Half the recipes in the book you're holding in your hands right now are built from ideas of Madison's; *Vegetarian Cooking* is a treasure trove of great recipes, a compendium of necessary techniques, and a fantastic source of inspiration. (She has also written *Vegetarian Suppers from Deborah Madison's Kitchen*, featuring simple preparations; *Local Flavors*, with a farmers market focus; and *This Can't Be Tofu!*, which is about...duh. All her books are fantastic, but the more specialized ones do have a lot of overlap with *Vegetarian Cooking*, so if you're not a compulsive cookbook collector like, ahem, someone else we know, just get the big, comprehensive one.)

sourcing

No matter where you live, it can be a serious challenge to find good, convenient, affordable places to shop for high-quality fresh food. It's not too hard to find farmers markets on the web—and more and more towns and cities across the U.S. have at least one—but I wish I could easily point you to the neighborhood shop with the great bulk section where you can stock up on grains and spices for cheap. I wish every neighborhood of every city or town had as many resources as my mine. I know that's not reality, but these websites can help. But to find the best bulk section in town—buying from the bulk bins is key to affordable spices—the best thing to do is probably to ask everyone you know.

- Coop Directory Service (www.coopdirectory.org). This is a list rather than a searchable database, but the site has a great bonus with its info on what coops are, their history, tips on starting your own, and a lot more general food-, sustainability-, and budget-related stuff.

- *Eat Where You Live: How to Find and Enjoy Local and Sustainable Food No Matter Where You Live*, by Lou Hendrick (Skipstone). The title says it all, really. As a folksy (sometimes overly so) li'l primer on finding local food sources, gardening basics, easy preserving, and more, this book really could be listed in a few places in this chapter. But I think the sourcing section is most useful, as she gathers a ton of information all in one place. It's well worth the tiny bit of cute overload you may experience.

- Food Co-Op Directory (www.cooperativegrocer.coop/coops). Just what it sounds like. Part of an online magazine called *Cooperative Grocer.*
- LocalHarvest (www.localharvest.org). This site operates an online store, which is kinda weird and seems counter to the whole local idea, but the really great thing is its database of small farms, farmers markets, and CSAs, which shows you where to get fresh local produce in your area. Don't use it for grocery stores, though; it's just not very complete.
- USDA's farmers market search (http://apps.ams.usda.gov/FarmersMarkets). Make sure you clear out the "<enter search criteria here>" text from the fields you're not using, or else your search won't return anything.

gardening

You might be asking yourself why I haven't talked much in this book about growing your own food. If you knew me well enough to know about my alarming lack of gardening skills, you wouldn't need to wonder. But gardening is, of course, a great way to produce fresh, extremely local food in an economical way (especially if your thumb is green enough to start plants from seed and you have a healthy compost bin). So I enlisted my community to help me with this section. Please don't blame Beth Alltop, Patricia Makins, Thisbe Nissen, Lisa Pimental, and Ivy Schlegel for any flaws or misinformation, though. That would be all mine.

- *Encyclopedia of Organic Gardening,* by J.I. Rodale and staff (Rodale Books). Originally published in 1959, it's been updated many times, most recently as *Rodale's All-New Encyclopedia of Organic Gardening: The Indispensable Resource for Every Gardener.*

Patricia says to get the original version, as it's more comprehensive than the new one. Full of indispensable overview information.

- *Four-Season Harvest: Organic Vegetables from Your Home Garden All Year Long*, by Eliot Coleman (Chelsea Green). Okay, Ivy recommended Coleman's other book, *The New Organic Grower*, but that one is more geared toward multiacre plots and producing enough to market–and if that's where you're at, you probably know way more than I do about what books to read. For the beginner, *Four-Season Harvest* seems more appropriate. Coleman lives in Maine and grows food year-round using simple cold frames. Sounds pretty awesome. Ivy says to expect a "down-home folksy feel."

- *Gaia's Garden: A Guide to Home-Scale Permaculture*, by Toby Hemenway (Chelsea Green). Beth recommended this one, and its online reviewers tend to use the word "bible" all the time and rave that it's the single most useful gardening book they have ever bought.

- *The Gardener's Table: A Guide to Natural Vegetable Growing and Cooking*, by Richard Merrill and Joe Ortiz (Ten Speed Press). In the interest of full disclosure, Ivy notes that one of the authors is a former professor of hers, and says, "This book is nice because it is organized by vegetable, is very conversationally written, and includes information on both growing and eating, which is a great combination."

- *The New Kitchen Garden*, by Anna Pavord (Dorling Kindersley). "Maybe DK books just please me aesthetically?" wonders Thisbe, but the food-growing focus here means that even if it's not comprehensive, it's still a good bet.

- *The Organic Garden Book*, by Geoff Hamilton (Dorling Kindersley). This was another one mentioned repeatedly by my panel of gardening experts because it's "the one I actually *use*" and it has "good demonstrations and illustrations."

- *Organic Gardening* (www.organicgardening.com). Lisa P., source of the spice rub on page 89, says her subscription to this magazine is invaluable. Plus, their website is extensive and well-organized.

- *The Sunset Western Garden Book* (Sunset Books). Every single Western-U.S. dweller who gave me suggestions mentioned this. Since Sunset is a West Coast company, unfortunately there is no Eastern analogue, but if you live in an area it covers, apparently you need this book. "I use this all the time, it's great for knowing what conditions plants need and when/where you should plant things based on your specific climate/location," says Patricia. Ivy adds, "Sunset's zone maps are better than the USDA zone maps because they account for discrete variations based on elevation, wind patterns, proximity to the sea, etc. There are thousands of other reasons why I love this book, but you don't need them all." So there.

- You Grow Girl (www.yougrowgirl.com). This is not the most well-organized site for a beginner (blog tags are not the way to present information that needs to be learned in an organized way), but there are active forums where you can get advice and exchange tips. If I were going to start a garden I think I would be hanging out there a lot.

- Your local county extension office (do a Google search for "gardening extension [the name of your county]"). Beth says, "First, all folks interested in gardening should know that every county in the U.S. should (in theory) have a county extension office offering *free* information and help growing plants and dealing with problem pests specific to that region. They were set up after the Civil

War when the land grant universities were established. Each county should also have a free hotline answered by people trained as Master Gardeners through an extension program that gives more thorough training for a very nominal fee; anyone can call in and ask any kind of gardening question." Sounds pretty great, yes?

canning and preserving

It's easy to think of home preserving as old-fashioned and no longer necessary, but it's actually a one of the best tools in any arsenal for year-round local eating. And now that we all have freezers at our disposal, the possibilities for saving your summer produce and eating it in January are greatly expanded, even for those who don't feel up to the task of spending the day canning. Though, I have to say, canning is a really fun activity when you get a group of friends together, and it's also great source of affordable gifts (who doesn't love a jar of homemade jam or tomato sauce?).

• The National Center for Home Food Preservation (www.uga. edu/nchfp). A project of the University of Georgia and a few other colleges, the NCHFP's mission is to provide food safety and preserving information, and research into innovations in the field. They've got publications such as *So Easy to Preserve*, a free online class, how-to sections for every kind of preserving, and a bunch of FAQs and seasonal tips with useful information, from the general (does freezing kill germs?) to the very specific (a recipe for spicy pumpkin leather).

• *Putting Food By*, by Janet Greene, Ruth Hertzberg, and Beatrice Vaughn (Plume). Beth recommended this one, and though I haven't read it myself it does seem like an incredibly useful resource. I think I'll get myself a copy sometime before next summer.

- PreserveFood.com (www.preservefood.com). This site provides a useful overview of different preserving methods (canning, drying, and freezing), the equipment you need, and a few recipes. It's basic, but that's what makes it good, especially if you're new to preserving. Bypass the vacuum sealing section, as a) they do seem to be shilling for a specific company and b) are you really going to buy and use a set of vacuum sealing equipment?

- *Wild Fermentation*, by Sandor Ellix Katz (Chelsea Green) and its companion website, www.wildfermentation.com. Okay, so fermentation isn't strictly a preservation technique, but making sauerkraut does make your head of cabbage last a lot longer. And all the stuff you can do with wild yeasts is rilly rilly cool, and Katz is so great himself (see *The Revolution Will Not Be Microwaved* in the Reading section above) that I can't resist the recommendation. Whether you're a food-chemistry geek, want to make your own tempeh/beer/sourdough, or just want to read about it, *Wild Fermentation* is for you.

activism

Here are some organizations working on food politics issues from community access to federal policy advocacy. Each can lead you to many more. Do I need to keep saying that these lists are not exhaustive?

- ALBA (www.albafarmers.org). Spelled out as the Agriculture and Land-Based Training Association (I guess the T would mess up the acronym too much), ALBA's mission is "to advance economic viability, social equity and ecological land management among limited-resource and aspiring farmers [and] to contribute to a more just and sustainable food system through the development of: 1) human resources that will be tomorrow's farmers and sustainable agriculture leaders; 2) growing marketing alternatives for small-scale, limited-resource farmers; and 3) the enhancement of biological diversity and protection of natural resources."

• Food First/Institute for Food and Development Policy (www. foodfirst.org). Focused on food sovereignty, local food systems, and land reform, Food First's mission is "to end the injustices that cause hunger, poverty and environmental degradation throughout the world."

• Growing Power (www.growingpower.org). This Milwaukee- and Chicago-based nonprofit grows food, trains youth in organic farming and micro-enterprise development, and educates community members about sustainable food systems.

• Healthy Corner Stores Network (www.healthycornerstores. org). An umbrella program for community groups, farmers, and public health departments working to get healthier food into the corner stores that serve as grocery stores in underserved neighborhoods.

• Midwest Organic and Sustainable Education Service (www. mosesorganic.org). MOSES's mission is "to help agriculture make the transition to a sustainable organic system of farming that is ecologically sound, economically viable, and socially just, through information, education, research, and integrating the broader community into this effort." The Organic Directory section of their website is especially helpful to the casual browser, with links to tons of other regional, national, and international organizations.

• The National Campaign for Sustainable Agriculture (www. sustainableagriculture.net). An education and outreach organization that "shape[s] and promote[s] federal agriculture policies that: support sound environmental stewardship and agriculture based economic development that is good for farm and ranch families and their communities, give consumers real choice about how their food is produced, [and] promote social justice and humane practices."

• The People's Grocery (www.peoplesgrocery.org). This awesome grassroots food justice group provides fresh, healthy food to residents of the low-income, totally-unserved-by-grocery-stores San Francisco Bay Area neighborhood of West Oakland, through urban gardening, a $12 CSA box, and more (they're working on opening a retail store).

• The Sustainable Agriculture Coalition (www.sustainableagriculturecoalition.org). With a membership ranging from ALBA, mentioned above, to the Union of Concerned Scientists, the coalition "advocate[s] for federal policies and programs supporting the long-term economic and environmental sustainability of agriculture, natural resources, and rural communities."

acknowledgments

SO MANY PEOPLE WERE INVOLVED IN THE MAKING OF THIS BOOK. I owe an enormous debt of gratitude to Debbie Rasmussen for, well, everything. Kick-starting and supporting my interest in whole foods is really the least of it, but it's the most relevant to this book: Without the many practical and political discussions she and I have had about food, I don't think I ever would have written it. (The other practical and political discussions we've had will work their way into the next book, I'm sure.)

A huge thanks to all my friends who inspired, donated ideas to, ate and critiqued the results of, and made suggestions to improve my recipes: Ann Marie Dobosz, Esti Feller, Erin Flaherty, Rachel Gratz, Mavis Gruver, Erik Hopp, Maya Phillipson, Lisa Pimental, Colin Sagan, Eleanor Sananman, Erin Siegel, and Christina Stork. (And thanks for being so much fun to cook for and eat with!)

Jen Angel and Janet Miller not only ate and critiqued with me but also lent me their sharp editorial eyes (and cooking expertise and curiosity, respectively); you, luckily, get to read the much-improved product of their suggestions instead of the originals.

I wouldn't have been able to write a complete resource section without gardening input from Beth Alltop, Patricia Makins, Thisbe Nissen, and Ivy Schlegel.

Thanks also go to Robb Kane and Ann Marie Powers for brainstorming a title (even though I changed it), Brian Awehali for making me a bet, Dixie de la Tour for listening to me yammering on about deglazing without putting a fork in my eye, Ben Shaykin for being a kick-ass designer who's willing to work for much less than he is worth, all the cookbook authors and food writers who don't know me from a turnip truck but who've taught me so much of what I'm passing along here, and everyone else I may have forgotten, for all the cool things they did.

Much appreciation to Ramsey Kanaan for taking a chance and letting me write whatever I wanted on the basis of one meeting and a follow-up e-mail.

No thank-yous would be complete without my parents, Bob and Kathe Jervis. This would be true even if it hadn't been my mother who taught me how to cook in the first place, because they have both supported me unflaggingly throughout every project I have ever taken on.

about the author

LISA JERVIS IS THE FOUNDING EDITOR AND PUBLISHER OF *BITCH:*
Feminist Response to Pop Culture, the founding board president of Women
in Media and News, and a member of the advisory board of outLoud Radio.
She is currently the finance and operations director at the Center for Media
Justice. Her work has appeared in numerous magazines and books, includ-
ing *Ms.*, the *San Francisco Chronicle*, *Utne*, *Mother Jones*, the *Women's
Review of Books*, *Bust*, the late and much-lamented *Hues*, *Salon*, the late
and also-lamented *Punk Planet*, *Body Outlaws* (Seal Press), *Tipping the
Sacred Cow* (AK Press) (a collection of writings from the late and lamented-
by-the-few-people-who've-heard-of-it *LiP: Informed Revolt*), and *The Bust
Guide to the New Girl Order* (Penguin). She is the coeditor of *Young
Wives' Tales: New Adventures in Love and Partnership* (Seal Press) and
Bitchfest: Ten Years of Cultural Criticism from the Pages of Bitch *Magazine.* She may someday get back to writing that long-planned book about
the intellectual legacy of gender essentialism and its effect on contem-
porary feminism. Having grown up in New York City, she retains a certain hard-nosed East Coast temperament, though the transplant to Oakland, California, has worked out remarkably well. In her spare time, she
squeezes fruit at farmer's markets, bikes around town, and tries not to
indulge her crazy-cat-lady tendencies too much.

about pm press

PM PRESS WAS FOUNDED AT THE END OF 2007 BY A SMALL collection of folks with decades of publishing, media, and organizing experience. PM cofounder Ramsey Kanaan started AK Press as a young teenager in Scotland almost 30 years ago and, together with his fellow PM Press coconspirators, has published and distributed hundreds of books, pamphlets, CDs, and DVDs. Members of PM have founded enduring book fairs, spearheaded victorious tenant organizing campaigns, and worked closely with bookstores, academic conferences, and even rock bands to deliver political and challenging ideas to all walks of life. We're old enough to know what we're doing and young enough to know what's at stake.

We seek to create radical and stimulating fiction and nonfiction books, pamphlets, t-shirts, and visual and audio materials to entertain, educate, and inspire you. We aim to distribute these through every available channel with every available technology—whether that means you are seeing anarchist classics at our bookfair stalls, reading our latest vegan cookbook at the café, downloading geeky fiction e-books, or digging new music and timely videos from our website.

PM Press is always on the lookout for talented and skilled volunteers, artists, activists, and writers to work with. If you have a great idea for a project or can contribute in some way, please get in touch.

PM Press

PO Box 23912

Oakland, CA 94623

www.pmpress.org

friends of pm

THESE ARE INDISPUTABLY MOMENTOUS TIMES—THE FINANCIAL system is melting down globally and the Empire is stumbling. Now more than ever there is a vital need for radical ideas.

In the year since its founding—and on a mere shoestring—PM Press has risen to the formidable challenge of publishing and distributing knowledge and entertainment for the struggles ahead. We have published an impressive and stimulating array of literature, art, music, politics, and culture. Using every available medium, we've succeeded in connecting those hungry for ideas and information to those putting them into practice.

Friends of PM allows you to directly help impact, amplify, and revitalize the discourse and actions of radical writers, filmmakers, and artists. It provides us with a stable foundation from which we can build upon our early successes and provides a much-needed subsidy for the materials that can't necessarily pay their own way.

It's a bargain for you too. For a minimum of $25 a month, you'll get all the audio and video (over a dozen CDs and DVDs in our first year) or all of the print releases (also over a dozen in our first year). For $40 you'll get everything that is published in hard copy. *Friends* also have the ability to purchase any/all items from our webstore at a 50% discount. And what could be better than the thrill of receiving a monthly package of cutting-edge political theory, art, literature, ideas, and practice delivered to your door?

Your card will be billed once a month, until you tell us to stop. Or until our efforts succeed in bringing the revolution around. Or the financial meltdown of Capital makes plastic redundant. Whichever comes first.

For more information on the *Friends of PM*, and about sponsoring particular projects, please go to www.pmpress.org, or contact us at info@pmpress.org.